KU-054-444

LIVERPOOL JMU LIBRARY

3 1111 01272 3308

Essential Statistics for the Pharmaceutical Sciences

Essential Statistics for the Pharmaceutical Sciences

Philip Rowe

Liverpool John Moores University, UK

BICENTENNIAL
1807
WILEY
2007
BICENTENNIAL

Copyright © 2007   John Wiley & Sons Ltd, The Atrium, Southern Gate, Chichester,
West Sussex PO19 8SQ, England

Telephone (+44) 1243 779777

Email (for orders and customer service enquiries): cs-books@wiley.co.uk
Visit our Home Page on www.wileyeurope.com or www.wiley.com

All Rights Reserved. No part of this publication may be reproduced, stored in a retrieval system or
transmitted in any form or by any means, electronic, mechanical, photocopying, recording, scanning or
otherwise, except under the terms of the Copyright, Designs and Patents Act 1988 or under the terms of
a licence issued by the Copyright Licensing Agency Ltd, 90 Tottenham Court Road, London W1T 4LP, UK,
without the permission in writing of the Publisher. Requests to the Publisher should be addressed to the
Permissions Department, John Wiley & Sons Ltd, The Atrium, Southern Gate, Chichester, West Sussex
PO19 8SQ, England, or emailed to permreq@wiley.co.uk, or faxed to (+44) 1243 770620.

Designations used by companies to distinguish their products are often claimed as trademarks.
All brand names and product names used in this book are trade names, service marks,
trademarks or registered trademarks of their respective owners. The Publisher is not associated
with any product or vendor mentioned in this book.

This publication is designed to provide accurate and authoritative information in regard to the subject
matter covered. It is sold on the understanding that the Publisher is not engaged in rendering
professional services. If professional advice or other expert assistance is required, the services of a
competent professional should be sought.

Other Wiley Editorial Offices

John Wiley & Sons Inc., 111 River Street, Hoboken, NJ 07030, USA
Jossey-Bass, 989 Market Street, San Francisco, CA 94103-1741, USA
Wiley-VCH Verlag GmbH, Boschstr. 12, D-69469 Weinheim, Germany
John Wiley & Sons Australia Ltd, 33 Park Road, Milton, Queensland 4064, Australia
John Wiley & Sons (Asia) Pte Ltd, 2 Clementi Loop #02-01, Jin Xing Distripark, Singapore 129809
John Wiley & Sons Canada Ltd, 6045 Freemont Blvd, Mississauga, Ontario, L5R 4J3

Wiley also publishes its books in a variety of electronic formats. Some content that appears in print may not
be available in electronic books.

Anniversary Logo Design: Richard J. Pacifico

Library of Congress Cataloguing-in-Publication Data

Rowe, Philip.
    Essential statistics for the pharmaceutical sciences / Philip Rowe.
       p. ; cm.
    Includes bibliographical references and index.
    ISBN-13: 978-0-470-03470-5 (cloth : alk. paper)
    ISBN-13: 978-0-470-03468-2 (pbk. : alk. paper)
  1. Drugs–Research–Statistical methods. 2.   Pharmacology–Statistical
methods. I. Title.
    [DNLM: 1. Pharmacology–methods. 2.   Statistics.   QV 20.5 R879e 2007]
    RS57.R69 2007
    615'.1072–dc22   2006102028

British Library Cataloguing in Publication Data

A catalogue record for this book is available from the British Library

ISBN-13: 978 0-470-03470-5 (HB)
ISBN-13: 978 0-470-03468-2 (PB)

Typeset in 10.5/12.5pt Minion by Thomson Digital
Printed in Great Britain by Antony Rowe Ltd., Chippenham, Wiltshire
This book is printed on acid-free paper responsibly manufactured from sustainable forestry
in which at least two trees are planted for each one used for paper production.

To

Carol, Joshua and Nathan

Contents

Preface   xiii

Statistical packages   xix

PART 1: DATA TYPES   1

1 Data types   3
  1.1 Does it really matter?   3
  1.2 Interval scale data   4
  1.3 Ordinal scale data   4
  1.4 Nominal scale data   5
  1.5 Structure of this book   6
  1.6 Chapter summary   6

PART 2: INTERVAL-SCALE DATA   7

2 Descriptive statistics   9
  2.1 Summarizing data sets   9
  2.2 Indicators of central tendency – mean, median and mode   10
  2.3 Describing variability – standard deviation and coefficient
      of variation   16
  2.4 Quartiles – another way to describe data   20
  2.5 Using computer packages to generate descriptive statistics   23
  2.6 Chapter summary   25

3 The normal distribution   27
  3.1 What is a normal distribution?   27
  3.2 Identifying data that are not normally distributed   28
  3.3 Proportions of individuals within one or two standard
      deviations of the mean   31
  3.4 Chapter summary   34

4 Sampling from populations – the SEM   35
  4.1 Samples and populations   35
  4.2 From sample to population   36
  4.3 Types of sampling error   37
  4.4 What factors control the extent of random sampling error?   39

	4.5	Estimating likely sampling error – The SEM	42
	4.6	Offsetting sample size against standard deviation	46
	4.7	Chapter summary	46

5 Ninety-five per cent confidence interval for the mean   **49**

	5.1	What is a confidence interval?	50
	5.2	How wide should the interval be?	50
	5.3	What do we mean by '95 per cent' confidence?	51
	5.4	Calculating the interval width	52
	5.5	A long series of samples and 95 per cent confidence intervals	53
	5.6	How sensitive is the width of the confidence interval to changes in the SD, the sample size or the required level of confidence?	54
	5.7	Two statements	56
	5.8	One-sided 95 per cent confidence intervals	57
	5.9	The 95 per cent confidence interval for the difference between two treatments	60
	5.10	The need for data to follow a normal distribution and data transformation	61
	5.11	Chapter summary	65

6 The two-sample *t*-test (1). Introducing hypothesis tests   **67**

	6.1	The two sample *t*-test – an example of a hypothesis test	68
	6.2	'Significance'	74
	6.3	The risk of a false positive finding	75
	6.4	What factors will influence whether or not we obtain a significant outcome?	76
	6.5	Requirements for applying a two-sample *t*-test	79
	6.6	Chapter summary	80

7 The two-sample *t*-test (2). The dreaded *P* value   **83**

	7.1	Measuring how significant a result is	83
	7.2	*P* values	84
	7.3	Two ways to define significance?	85
	7.4	Obtaining the *P* value	86
	7.5	*P* values or 95 per cent confidence intervals?	86
	7.6	Chapter summary	87

8 The two-sample *t*-test (3). False negatives, power and necessary sample sizes   **89**

	8.1	What else could possibly go wrong?	90
	8.2	Power	91
	8.3	Calculating necessary sample size	94
	8.4	Chapter summary	101

9 The two-sample *t*-test (4). Statistical significance, practical significance and equivalence   **103**

| | 9.1 | Practical significance – is the difference big enough to matter? | 104 |

9.2	Equivalence testing	107
9.3	Non-inferiority testing	111
9.4	*P* values are less informative and can be positively misleading	113
9.5	Setting equivalence limits prior to experimentation	115
9.6	Chapter summary	116

10 The two-sample *t*-test (5). One-sided testing   117

10.1	Looking for a change in a specified direction	118
10.2	Protection against false positives	120
10.3	Temptation!	121
10.4	Using a computer package to carry out a one-sided test	125
10.5	Should one-sided tests be used more commonly?	126
10.5	Chapter summary	126

11 What does a statistically significant result really tell us?   127

11.1	Interpreting statistical significance	127
11.2	Starting from extreme scepticism	131
11.3	Chapter summary	132

12 The paired *t*-test – comparing two related sets of measurements   133

12.1	Paired data	133
12.2	We could analyse the data using a two-sample *t*-test	135
12.3	Using a paired *t*-test instead	135
12.4	Performing a paired *t*-test	136
12.5	What determines whether a paired *t*-test will be significant?	138
12.6	Greater power of the paired *t*-test	139
12.7	The paired *t*-test is only applicable to naturally paired data	139
12.8	Choice of experimental design	140
12.9	Requirements for applying a paired *t*-test	141
12.10	Sample sizes, practical significance and one-sided tests	141
12.11	Summarizing the differences between the paired and two-sample *t*-tests	143
12.12	Chapter summary	144

13 Analyses of variance – going beyond *t*-tests   145

13.1	Extending the complexity of experimental designs	146
13.2	One-way analysis of variance	146
13.3	Two-way analysis of variance	156
13.4	Multi-factorial experiments	164
13.5	Keep it simple – Keep it powerful	165
13.6	Chapter summary	167

14 Correlation and regression – relationships between measured values   169

14.1	Correlation analysis	170
14.2	Regression analysis	178

14.3 Multiple regression   185
14.4 Chapter summary   192

PART 3: NOMINAL-SCALE DATA   195

15 Describing categorized data   197
15.1 Descriptive statistics   198
15.2 Testing whether the population proportion might credibly
      be some pre-determined figure   202
15.3 Chapter summary   207

16 Comparing observed proportions – the contingency
      chi-square test   209
16.1 Using the contingency chi-square test to compare
      observed proportions   210
16.2 Obtaining a 95 per cent CI for the change in the proportion of
      expulsions – is the difference large enough to be of practical
      significance?   213
16.3 Larger tables – attendance at diabetic clinics   214
16.4 Planning experimental size   217
16.5 Chapter summary   219

PART 4: ORDINAL-SCALE DATA   221

17 Ordinal and non-normally distributed data. Transformations
      and non-parametric tests   223
17.1 Transforming data to a normal distribution   224
17.2 The Mann–Whitney test – a non-parametric method   228
17.3 Dealing with ordinal data   233
17.4 Other non-parametric methods   235
17.5 Chapter summary   242
      Appendix to chapter 17   242

PART 5: SOME CHALLENGES FROM THE REAL WORLD   245

18 Multiple testing   247
18.1 What is it and why is it a problem?   247
18.2 Where does multiple testing arise?   248
18.3 Methods to avoid false positives   250
18.4 The role of scientific journals   254
18.5 Chapter summary   255

19 Questionnaires   257
19.1 Is there anything special about questionnaires?   258
19.2 Types of questions   258
19.3 Designing a questionnaire   262
19.4 Sample sizes and return rates   263

19.5   Analysing the results   265
19.6   Confounded epidemiological data   266
19.7   Multiple testing with questionnaire data   271
19.8   Chapter summary   272

PART 6: CONCLUSIONS   **275**

20   Conclusions   **277**
20.1   Be clear about the purpose of the experiment   277
20.2   Keep the experimental design simple and therefore
      clear and powerful   278
20.3   Draw up a statistical analysis plan as part of the experimental
      design – it is not a last minute add-on   279
20.4   Explore your data visually before launching into
      statistical testing   280
20.5   Beware of multiple analyses   281
20.6   Interpret both significance and non-significance with care   282

Index   **283**

Preface

At whom is this book aimed?

Statistics users rather than statisticians

As a subject, statistics is boring, irrelevant and incomprehensible. Well, traditionally it is anyway. The subject does not have to be that bad; It simply has not escaped from a self-imposed time-warp. Thirty years ago, there were no easy-to-use computer packages that would do all the hard sums for us. So, inevitably, the subject was heavily bogged down in the 'How to' questions – how do we most efficiently calculate the average weight of 500 potatoes? How do we work out whether the yield of turnips really did increase when we used a couple of extra shovels of horse manure? How should we calculate whether there really is a relationship between rainfall and the size of our apples? Thirty years ago, statistical authors had a genuine excuse for their books being clogged up with detailed methods of calculation. However, one might ask, what is their excuse today? Nowadays, nobody in their right mind would manually calculate a complex statistical test, so why do they still insist on telling us how to do it?

Clearly the world does need genuine 'statisticians' to maintain and improve analytical methods and such people do need to understand the detailed working of specific procedures. However, the majority of us are not statisticians as such; we just want to use statistical methods to achieve a particular end. We should be distinguishing between 'statisticians' and 'statistics users'. It is rather like the distinction between automotive engineers and motorists. Automotive engineering is an honourable and necessary profession, but most of us are just simple motorists. Fortunately, within the field of motoring, the literature does respect the difference. If a book is written for motorists, it will simply tell us that, if we want to go faster, we should press the accelerator. It will not bore us stiff trying to explain how the fuel injection system achieves that particular end. Unfortunately that logic has never crept into statistics books. The wretched things still insist on trying to explain the internal workings of the Kolmogorov–Smirnov test to an audience who could not care less.

Well, good news! This book is quite happy to treat any statistical calculation as a black box. It will explain what needs to go into the box and it will explain what comes out the other end, but you can remain as ignorant about what goes on inside the box as you are about how your power steering works. This approach is not just lazy or negative. By stripping away all the irrelevant bits, we can focus on the aspects that actually matter. This book will try to concentrate on those issues that statistics users really do need to understand:

- Why are statistical procedures necessary at all?

- How can statistics help in planning experiments?

- Which procedure should I employ to analyse the results?

- What do the statistical results actually mean when I have got them?

Who are these 'statistics users'?

The people that this book is aimed at are those thousands of people who have to use statistical procedures without having any ambition to become statisticians. There are any number of student programmes, ranging from pharmacology and botany through to business studies and psychology, which will include an element of statistics. These students will have to learn to use at least the more basic statistical methods. There are also those of us engaged in research in academia or industry. Some of us will have to carry out our own statistical analyses and others will be able to call on the services of professional statisticians. However, even where professionals are to hand, there is still the problem of communication. If you do not even know what the words mean, you are going to have great difficulty explaining to a statistician exactly what you want to do. The intention is that all of the above should find this book useful.

If you are a statistics student or a professional statistician, my advice would be to put this book down now! You will probably find its dismissive attitude towards the mathematical basis of your trade extremely irritating. Indeed, if at least one traditional statistician does not complain bitterly about this book, I shall be rather disappointed.

To what subject area is the book relevant?

All the statistical procedures and tests mentioned are illustrated with practical examples and data sets. The cases are drawn from the pharmaceutical sciences and this is reflected in the book's title. However, pretty well all the methods described and the principles explored are perfectly relevant to a wide range of scientific research, including pharmaceutical, biological, biomedical and chemical sciences.

At what level is it aimed?

The book is aimed at undergraduate science students and their teachers and less experienced researchers.

The early chapters (1–5) are fairly basic. They cover data description (mean, median, mode, standard deviation and quartile values) and introduce the problem of describing uncertainty due to sampling error (SEM and 95 per cent confidence interval for the mean). In theory, much of this should be familiar from secondary education, but in the author's experience, the reality is that many new students cannot (for example) calculate the median for a small data set. These chapters are therefore relevant to level 1 students, for either teaching or revision purposes.

Chapters 6–17 then cover the most commonly used statistical tests. Most undergraduate programmes will introduce such material fairly early on (levels 1 or 2). The approach used is not the traditional one of giving equal weight to a wide range of techniques. As the focus of the book is the various issues surrounding statistical testing rather than methods of calculation, one test (the two-sample t-test) has been used to illustrate all the relevant issues (Chapters 6–11). Further chapters (12–17) then deal with other tests more briefly, referring back to principles that have now been established.

The final chapters (18 and 19) cover some real-world problems that students probably will not run into until their final year, when carrying out their own independent research projects. The issues considered are multiple testing (all too common in student projects!) and questionnaire design and analysis. While the latter does not introduce many fundamentally new concepts, the use of questionnaires has increased so much, it seemed useful to bring together all the relevant points in a single resource.

Key point and pirate boxes

Key point boxes

Throughout the book you will find key point boxes that look like this:

⚷ Proportions of individuals within given ranges

For data that follow a normal distribution:

- about two-thirds of individuals will have values within 1 SD of the mean;

- about 95 per cent of individuals will have values within 2 SD of the mean.

These never provide new information. Their purpose is to summarize and emphasize key points.

Pirate boxes

You will also find pirate boxes that look like this:

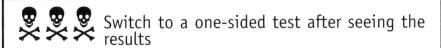 Switch to a one-sided test after seeing the results

Even today, this is probably the best and most commonly used statistical fiddle.

You did the experiment and analysed the results by your usual two-sided test. The result fell just short of significance (*P* somewhere between 0.05 and 0.1) There is a simple solution, guaranteed to work every time. Re-run the analysis, but change to a one-sided test, testing for a change in whatever direction you now know the results actually suggest.

Until the main scientific journals get their act into gear, and start insisting that authors register their intentions in advance, there is no way to detect this excellent fiddle. You just need some plausible reason why you 'always intended' to do a one-tailed test in this particular direction, and you are guaranteed to get away with it.

These are written in the style of Machiavelli, but are not actually intended to encourage statistical abuse. The point is to make you alert for misuses that others may try to foist upon you. Forewarned is forearmed. The danger posed is reflected by the number of skull and cross-bone symbols.

Minor hazard. Abuse easy to spot or has limited potential to mislead.

Moderate hazard. The well-informed (e.g. readers of this book) should spot the attempted deception.

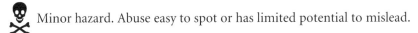 Severe hazard. An effective ruse that even the best informed may suspect, but never be able to prove.

Fictitious data

Throughout this book, all the experiments described are entirely fictitious as are their results. Generally the structure of the experiments and the results are realistic. In a few cases, both the structure of an experiment and consequently the analysis of the results may be somewhat simpler than would often be seen in the real world. Clarity seems more important than strict realism.

At several points, judgements are quoted as to how greatly a measured end-point would need to change, for that change to be of any practical consequence. The values quoted are essentially arbitrary, being something that appears realistic to the author. Hopefully these are reasonable estimates, but none of them should be viewed as expert opinion.

A potted summary of this book

The book is aimed at those who have to use statistics, but have no ambition to become statisticians *per se*. It avoids getting bogged down in calculation methods and focuses instead on crucial issues that surround data generation and analysis (sample size estimation, interpretation of statistical results, the hazards of multiple testing, potential abuses, etc.). In this day of statistical packages, it is the latter that cause the real problems, not the number-crunching.

The book's illustrative examples are all taken from the pharmaceutical sciences, so students (and staff) in the areas of pharmacy, pharmacology and pharmaceutical science should feel at home with all the material. However, the issues considered are of concern in most scientific disciplines and should be perfectly clear to anybody from a similar discipline, even if the examples are not immediately familiar. Material is arranged in a developmental manner. Initial chapters are aimed at level 1 students; this material is fairly basic, with special emphasis on random sampling error. The next section then covers key concepts that may be introduced at levels 1 or 2. The final couple of chapters are most likely to be useful during final year research projects; These include one on questionnaire design and analysis.

The book is not tied to any specific statistical package. Instructions should allow readers to enter data into any package and find the key parts of the output. Specific instructions for performing all the procedures, using Minitab or SPSS, are provided in a linked web site (www.staff.ljmu.ac.uk/phaprowe/pharmstats.htm).

Statistical packages

There are any number of statistical packages available. It is not the intention of this book to recommend any particular package. Quite frankly, most of them are not worth recommending.

Microsoft XL

Probably the commonest way to collect data and perform simple manipulations is within a Microsoft XL spread-sheet. Consequently, the most obvious way to carry out statistical analyses of such data would seem to lie within XL itself. Let me give you my first piece of advice. Do not even consider it! The data analysis procedures within XL are rubbish – a very poor selection of procedures, badly implemented (apart from that, they are OK). If anybody in the Microsoft Corporation had a clue, they could have cleaned up in this area years ago. The opposition is pretty feeble and a decent statistical analysis package built into XL would have been unstoppable.

It is only at the most basic level that XL is of any real use (calculation of the mean, SD and SEM). It is therefore mentioned in some of the early chapters but not thereafter.

Other packages

A small survey by the author suggests that, in the subject areas mainly targetted by this book, only Minitab and SPSS are used with any frequency. Other packages seem to be restricted to very small numbers of departments. A decision was taken not to include blow-by-blow accounts of how to perform specific tests using any package, as this would excessively limit the book's audience. Instead, general comments are made about:

- entering data into packages;

- the information that will be required before any package can carry out the procedure;

- what to look for in the output that will be generated.

The last point is usually illustrated by generic output. This will not be in the same format as that from any specific package, but will present information that they should all provide.

Detailed instructions for Minitab and SPSS on the web site

As Minitab and SPSS clearly do have a significant user base, detailed instructions on how to use these packages to execute the procedures in this book, will be made available through the website associated with the book (www.staff.ljmu.ac.uk/phaprowe/pharmstats.htm). These cover how to:

- arrange the data for analysis;

- trigger the appropriate test;

- select appropriate options where relevant;

- find the essential parts of the output.

Part 1

Data types

1

Data types

This chapter will ...

- Set out a system for describing different types of data

- Explain why we need to identify the type of data we are dealing with

---

1.1 Does it really matter?

To open a statistics book with a discussion of the way in which data can be categorized into different types probably sounds horribly academic. However, the first step in selecting a data handling technique is generally identifying what type of data we are dealing with. So, it may be dry, but it does have real consequences.

We will look at three types of data. All of these go under a variety of names. I have chosen names that seem to me to be the most self-explanatory, rather than sticking rigorously to any consistent system. The three terms that I will use are:

- interval scale – continuous measurement data;

- ordinal scale – ordered categorical data;

- nominal scale – categorical data.

Essential Statistics for the Pharmaceutical Sciences   Philip Rowe
© 2007 John Wiley & Sons, Ltd   ISBN 9780 470 03470 5 (HB)   ISBN 9780 470 03468 2 (PB)

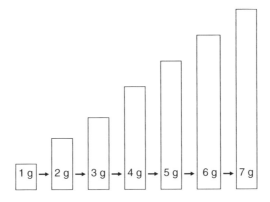

Figure 1.1 Interval scale data – a series of weights (1–7 g)

1.2 Interval scale data

The first two types of data that we will consider are both concerned with the measurement of some characteristic. 'Interval scale', or what is commonly called 'Continuous measurement', data include most of the information that would be generated in a laboratory. These include weights, lengths, timings, concentrations, pressures, etc. Imagine we had a series of objects weighing 1, 2, 3 up to 7 g as in Figure 1.1.

Now think about the differences in weights as we step from one object to the next. These steps, each of one unit along the scale, have the following characteristics:

1. *The steps are of an exactly defined size.* If you told somebody that you had a series of objects like those described above, he or she would know exactly how large the weight differences were as we progressed along the series.

2. *All the steps are of exactly the same size.* The weight difference between the 1 and 2 g objects is the same as the step from 2 to 3 g or from 6 to 7 g, and so on.

Because these measurements have constant sized steps (intervals), the measurement scale is described as a 'constant interval scale' and the data as 'interval scale'. Although the weights quoted in Figure 1.1 are exact integers, weights of 1.5 or 3.175 g are perfectly possible, so the measurement scale is said to be 'continuous'.

1.3 Ordinal scale data

Again measurement is involved, but the characteristic being assessed is often more subjective in nature. It is all well and good to measure nice neat objective things like blood pressure or temperature, but it is also a good idea to get the patient's angle on

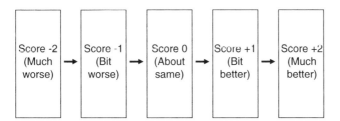

Figure 1.2 Ordinal scale data – scores for patient responses to treatment

how they feel about their treatment. The most obvious way to do this is as a score, of (say) −2 to +2 with the following equivalences:

$$-2 = \text{markedly worse}$$
$$-1 = \text{a bit worse}$$
$$0 = \text{about the same}$$
$$+1 = \text{a bit better}$$
$$+2 = \text{markedly better}$$

In this case (Figure 1.2), all we know is that, if one patient has a higher value than another, they are more satisfied with their outcome. However, we have no idea how much more satisfied he/she might be.

Since we have no idea how large the steps are between scores, we obviously cannot claim that all steps are of equal size. In fact, it is not even necessarily the case that the difference between scores of −2 and 0 is greater than that between +1 and +2. So, neither of the special characteristics of an constant interval scale apply to this data.

The name 'ordinal' reflects the fact that the various outcomes form an ordered sequence going from one extreme to its opposite. Such data are sometimes referred to as 'ordered categorical'. In this case the data are usually discontinuous, individual cases being scored as −1, +2 etc., with no fractional values.

1.4 Nominal scale data

In this case there is no sense of measuring a characteristic. With this data we use a system of classifications, with no natural ordering. For example, one of the factors that might influence the effectiveness of treatment could be the specific manufacturer of a medical device. Therefore, all patients would be classified as users of 'Smith', 'Jones' or 'Williams' equipment. There is no natural sequence to these; they are just three different makes.

With ordinal data we did at least know that a case scored as (say) +2 is going to be more similar to one scored +1 than to one scored 0 or −1. However, with nominal data, we have no reason to expect Smith or Jones equipment to have any special degree of similarity. Indeed the sequence in which one would list them may be entirely arbitrary.

Quite commonly there are just two categories in use. Obvious cases are male/female, alive/dead or success/failure. In these cases, the data are described as 'dichotomous'.

⚷ Data types

- *Interval scale* – measurements with defined and constant intervals between successive values. Values are continuous.

- *Ordinal scale* – measurements using classifications with a natural sequence (lowest to highest), but with undefined intervals. Values are discontinuous.

- *Nominal scale* – classifications that form no natural sequence.

1.5 Structure of this book

The structure of this book is based upon the different data types. Chapters 2–14 all deal with the handling of continuous measurement data, with Chapters 15 and 16 focusing on categorical data, and then Chapter 17 covers ordered data.

1.6 Chapter summary

When selecting statistical procedures, a vital first step is to identify the type of data that is being considered.

Data may be:

- *Interval scale* – measurements on a scale with defined and constant intervals. Data are continuous.

- *Ordinal scale* – measurements on a scale without defined intervals. Data are discontinuous.

- *Nominal scale* – classifications that form no natural sequence.

Part 2
Interval-scale data

2
Descriptive statistics

This chapter will . . .

- Review the use of the mean, median or mode to indicate how small or large a set of values is and consider when each is most appropriate

- Describe the use of the standard deviation to indicate how variable a set of values is

- Show how quartiles can be used to convey information similar to that mentioned above, even in the presence of extreme outlying values

---

2.1 Summarizing data sets

Experiments and trials frequently produce lists of figures that are too long to be easily comprehended and we need to produce one or two summary figures that will give the reader an accurate picture of the overall situation.

With interval scale (continuous measurement) data, there are two aspects to the figures that we should be trying to describe:

- How large are they?

- How variable are they?

Essential Statistics for the Pharmaceutical Sciences   Philip Rowe
© 2007 John Wiley & Sons, Ltd   ISBN 9780 470 03470 5 (HB)   ISBN 9780 470 03468 2 (PB)

To indicate the first of these, we quote an 'indicator of central tendency' and for the second an 'indicator of dispersion'.

In this chapter we look at more than one possible approach to both of the above. It would be wrong to claim that one way is universally better than another. However, we can make rational choices for specific situations if we take account of the nature of the data and the purpose of the report.

⚗️ Descriptive Statistics

Indicators of central tendency: how large are the numbers?
Indicators of dispersion: how variable are the numbers?

2.2 Indicators of central tendency – mean, median and mode

The term 'indicator of central tendency' describes any statistic that is used to indicate an average value around which the data are clustered. Three possible indicators of central tendency are in common use – the mean, median and mode.

2.2.1 Mean – 10 batches of vaccine

The usual approach to showing the central tendency of a set of data is to quote the average. However, academics abhor such terms as their meanings are far too well known. We naturally prefer something a little more obscure – the 'mean'.

Our first example set of data concerns a series of batches of vaccine. Each batch is intended to be of equal potency, but some manufacturing variability is unavoidable. A series of 10 batches has been analysed and the results are shown in Table 2.1.

Table 2.1 Potency of 10 batches of vaccine (units/ml)

	Potency (units/ml)
	106.6
	97.9
	102.3
	95.6
	93.6
	95.9
	101.8
	99.5
	94.9
	103.4
Mean = 99.15	

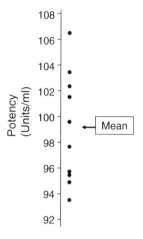

Figure 2.1 The mean satisfactorily indicates a typical potency among 10 batches of vaccine

The sum of all the potencies is 991.5 and dividing that by the number of observations (10) gives an average or mean activity of 99.15 units/ml.

The arithmetic is not open to serious question, but what we do need to consider is whether the figure we quote will convey an appropriate message to the reader. Although it may not strictly be justified, many readers will view that figure of 99.15 units/ml as indicating a typical figure. In other words, a batch with an activity of 99.15 units/ml is neither strikingly weak nor abnormally potent. A visual representation of the data is useful in testing whether this really is the case – see Figure 2.1.

The mean is nicely slap-bang in the middle of the bunch of values and does indicate a perfectly typical value. In this case the simple mean works fine and there is no need to consider more obscure alternatives. However, this is not always the case.

2.2.2 Median – time to open a child-proof container

Fifteen patients were provided with their drugs in a child-proof container of a design that they had not previously experienced. A note was taken of the time it took each patient to get the container open for the first time. The second column of Table 2.2 shows the results.

The mean is shown as 7.09 s, but again, we need to ask about the message that may be conveyed. Is this a representative figure? Figure 2.2 shows that it definitely is not.

Most patients have got the idea more or less straight away and have taken only 2–5 s to open the container. However, four seem to have got the wrong end of the stick and have ended up taking anything up to 25 s. These four have contributed a disproportionate amount of time (65.6 s) to the overall total. This has then increased the mean to 7.09 s. We would not consider a patient who took 7.09 s to be remotely typical. In fact they would be distinctly slow.

This problem of mean values being disproportionately affected by a minority of outliers arises quite frequently in biological and medical research. A useful approach

Table 2.2 Ranked times taken to open a child-proof container and calculation of the median

Rank	Time (s)	
1	2.2	
2	3.0	
3	3.1	
4	3.2	
5	3.4	
6	3.9	
7	4.0	
8	4.1 ←	The median value
9	4.2	
10	4.5	
11	5.1	
12	10.7	
13	12.2	
14	17.9	
15	24.8	
	Mean = 7.09 s	

is to use the median. To obtain this, the results shown in Table 2.2 are in ranked order (quickest at the top to slowest at the bottom) and their ranking positions are shown in the first column. We want to find the middle individual. This is the one ranked eighth, as there are seven patients slower and seven faster than this individual. The median is then the time taken by this eighth ranking individual, i.e. 4.1 s.

Figure 2.2 shows that a patient taking 4.1 s is genuinely typical. So, in this case, the median is a better indicator of a representative figure.

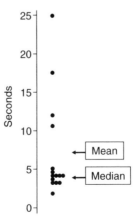

Figure 2.2 The median satisfactorily indicates a typical time taken to open a novel child-proof container. The mean is distorted by outliers

Should we automatically use the median in such cases? It would be an over-generalization to suggest that in every case where the data have outliers the median is automatically the statistic to quote. We need to keep an eye on what use is to be made of the information. If we were dealing with the cost of a set of items and the intention was to predict the cost of future sets of such items, the mean would be appropriate even if there were outliers. The only way to predict the cost of a future batch of items would be to multiply the number of items by our estimate of the mean individual cost. For those purposes, the median would be useless.

The median is robust to extreme outliers The term 'robust' is used to indicate that a statistic or a procedure will continue to give a reasonable outcome even if some of the data are aberrant. Think what would happen if the slow-coach who took 24.8 s to crack the child-proof container had instead taken a week to get it open. This character, who is currently ranked 15th, would still be ranked 15th and the median, which is established by the eighth ranker, would be quite unchanged at 4.1 s. In contrast, the mean would be hugely inflated if somebody took a week.

This resistance to the effects of a few silly values is the reason that the median is considered to be robust and the mean much less so.

In the right hands, this robustness is a useful characteristic and can allow us to indicate a representative figure even if a few bizarre figures have crept in. The danger is always that of potential abuse, where somebody wants to use the median to hide the embarrassing handful of cases that spoilt their otherwise beautiful set of results.

 ## The median

The middle ranking value. Especially useful with data containing occasional highly outlying values. It is 'robust' (resists the influence of aberrant data).

☠ ☠ Use the median to abolish those wretched outliers

Put this one up against a reasonably untutored readership and you should get away with it.

Simply quote the median for a group of observations, but make no mention of the outliers and under no circumstances publish the full set of individual results. That way, your median will be dominated by the majority of the data points and the outliers should nicely disappear from view.

Calculating the median where there is an even number of observations In the example above (Table 2.2), the total number of timings is 15. With any odd number

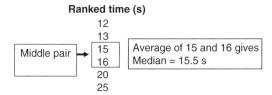

Figure 2.3   Calculation of a median with an even number of data points (timings in seconds)

of data points, we can identify a single middle-ranking individual. However, with even numbers of observations there is no middle individual. In those cases, we identify the middle pair and then use the average of their values. An example of six timings is shown in Figure 2.3.

One slightly awkward consequence is that, although the timings were apparently made to the nearest whole number of seconds, we can end up with a median value that contains a fraction.

2.2.3   Mode – a global assessment variable for the response to an anti-inflammatory drug

The condition of a series of patients with arthritis is recorded using a global assessment variable. This is a composite measure that takes account of both objective measures of the degree of inflammation of a patient's joints and subjective measures of the restrictions on their quality of life. It is set up so that higher scores represent better condition. The patients are then switched to a new anti-inflammatory product for 3 months and re-assessed using the same global measure. We then calculate the change in score for each individual. A positive score indicates an improvement and a negative one a deterioration in the patient's condition. Sixty patients participated and the results are shown in Table 2.3.

A histogram of the above data (Figure 2.4) shows the difficulty we are going to have. Most of the patients have shown reduced joint inflammation, but there are two distinct sub-populations so far as side effects are concerned. Slightly under half the patients are relatively free of side effects, so their quality of life improves markedly, but for the remainder, side effects are of such severity that their lives are actually made considerably worse overall.

Mathematically, it is perfectly possible to calculate a mean or a median among these score changes and these are shown on Figure 2.4. However, neither indicator remotely encapsulates the situation. The mean (-0.77) is particularly unhelpful as it indicates a value that is very untypical – very few patients show changes close to zero. We need to describe the fact that, in this case, there are two distinct groups.

The first two sets of data we looked at (vaccine potencies and container opening timings) consisted of values clustered around some single central point. Such data are referred to as 'unimodal'. The general term 'polymodal' is used for any case with

Table 2.3 Individual changes in a global assessment variable
following treatment with an anti-inflammatory (61 patients)

	Score changes	
11	−9	−8
0	−9	2
−5	−15	−11
11	−13	−12
−13	−13	10
7	−18	−11
7	−13	9
−12	9	14
10	14	−9
−12	10	17
−10	−9	−14
6	11	−6
13	−11	13
−11	14	12
10	10	−6
−9	21	−9
9	6	2
8	−13	5
−12	−6	−7
10	−9	−12
1		

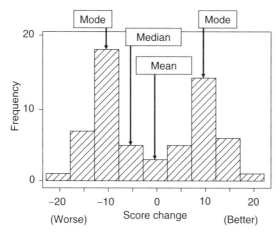

Figure 2.4 Individual changes in a global assessment score. Neither mean nor median
indicates a typical value with bimodal data. Only modes achieve this

several clusterings. If we want to be more precise, we use terms such as bimodal or trimodal to describe the exact number of clusters. The arthritis data might be described generally as polymodal or more specifically as bimodal.

With polymodal data we need to indicate the central tendency of each cluster. This is achieved by quoting the most commonly occurring value (the 'mode') within each cluster. For the arthritis data, the two modes are score changes of -10 and $+10$. We would therefore summarize the results as being bimodal with modes of -10 and $+10$.

🔑 **Unimodal and polymodal data**

Unimodal – in a single cluster.
Polymodal – in more than one cluster (a general term).
Bimodal – specifically in two clusters.
Trimodal – in three clusters, etc.

🔑 **The mode**

A value that occurs with peak frequency. The only effective way to describe polymodal data.

2.2.4 Selecting an indicator of central tendency

There is a definite pecking order among the three indicators of central tendency described above. The mean is the industry standard and is the most useful for a whole range of further purposes. Unless there are specific problems (e.g. polymodality or marked skewness), the mean is the indicator of choice. The median is met with pretty frequently and the mode (or modes) tends only to be used when all else fails.

2.3 Describing variability – standard deviation and coefficient of variation

2.3.1 Standard deviation

We have two tabletting machines producing erythromycin tablets with a nominal content of 250 mg. The two machines are made by the 'Alpha' and 'Bravo' Tabletting Machine Corporations, respectively. Five hundred tablets are randomly selected

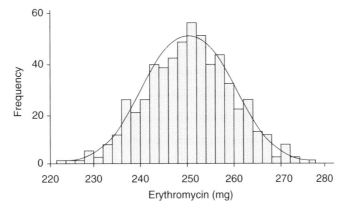

Figure 2.5 Histogram of erythromycin content of 500 tablets from an Alpha tabletting machine (relatively variable product – large standard deviation)

from each machine and their erythromycin contents assayed. The results for both machines are shown as histograms in Figures 2.5 and 2.6. To produce these histograms the drug contents have been categorized into bands 2 mg wide. (The curves superimposed onto the histograms are discussed in the next chapter.)

The two machines are very similar in terms of average drug content for the tablets, both producing tablets with a mean very close to 250 mg. However, the two products clearly differ. With the Alpha machine, there is a considerable proportion of tablets with a content differing by more than 10 mg from the nominal dose (i.e. below 240 mg or above 260 mg), whereas with the Bravo machine, such outliers are much rarer. An 'indicator of dispersion' is required in order to convey this difference in variability.

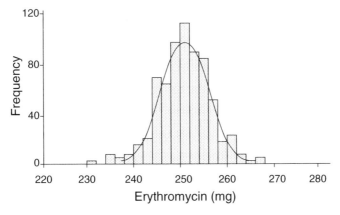

Figure 2.6 Histogram of erythromycin content of 500 tablets from a Bravo tabletting machine (more constant product – smaller standard deviation)

Table 2.4 Erythromycin contents of 10 tablets from an Alpha and a Bravo tabletting machine and calculation of their standard deviations

Alpha machine			Bravo machine		
Erythro content (mg)	Deviation from mean	Deviation squared	Erythro content (mg)	Deviation from mean	Deviation squared
249	0.3	0.09	251	−0.1	0.01
242	−6.7	44.89	247	−4.1	16.81
252	3.3	10.89	257	5.9	34.81
235	−13.7	187.69	250	−1.1	1.21
257	8.3	68.89	254	2.9	8.41
244	−4.7	22.09	251	−0.1	0.01
264	15.3	234.09	252	0.9	0.81
249	0.3	0.09	255	3.9	15.21
255	6.3	39.69	244	−7.1	50.41
240	−8.7	75.69	250	−1.1	1.21
Mean		Total	Mean		Total
248.7		684.1	251.1		128.9

Sum of squared deviations $= 684.1$
$684.1/9 = 76.01$
SD $=$ square root 76.01
   $= \mathbf{8.72\ mg\ (SD)}$

Sum of squared deviations $= 128.9$
$128.9/9 = 14.32$
SD $=$ square root 14.32
   $= \mathbf{3.78\ mg\ (SD)}$

The standard deviation (SD) is the most commonly accepted indicator of dispersion. This book generally discourages time-wasting manual calculations, but it is worth looking at an example of how the SD is calculated, because it makes clear what it reflects. The calculation of an SD for erythromycin content in samples of 10 tablets from the two machines is shown in Table 2.4. The first column shows the drug contents of 10 individual tablets from an Alpha machine. The mean among these is 248.7 mg. The next column then shows the 'deviation' of each individual tablet from the group mean. So, for example, the first tablet contained 249 mg of drug, which is 0.3 mg more than the average. Hence the figure of 0.3 in the next column. The details of the rest of the calculation are not wildly interesting, but are presented for completeness. The next step is to take all the individual deviations and square them as in the third column. We then sum these figures and obtain 684.1. That is then divided by the number of observations minus 1, yielding 76.01. Finally, we take the square root (8.72 mg) and that is the SD.

The key step in the calculation is the production of the second column – the individual deviations from the mean. The first machine produces rather variable tablets and so several of the tablets deviate considerably (e.g. −13.7 or +15.3 mg) from the overall mean. These relatively large figures then feed through the rest of the calculation, producing a high final SD (8.72 mg).

In contrast, the Bravo machine is more consistent and individual tablets never have a drug content much above or below the overall average. The small figures in the column of individual deviations then feed through the rest of the sausage machine, leading to a lower SD (3.78 mg).

Reporting the SD – the '±' symbol   The ± symbol – reasonably interpreted as meaning 'more or less' – is used to indicate variability. With the tablets from our two machines, we would report their drug contents as:

Alpha machine: 248.7 ± 8.72 mg (±SD)
Bravo machine: 251.1 ± 3.78 mg (±SD)

Since it is conceivable that some statistic other than the SD has been quoted, it is useful to state this explicitly. When a result is simply quoted as one figure ± another figure, we would normally assume that it is the SD that has been provided.

The figures quoted above succinctly summarize the true situation. The two machines produce tablets with almost identical mean contents, but those from the Alpha machine are two to three times more variable.

Units of SD   The SD is *not* a unitless number. It has the same units as the individual pieces of data. Since our data consisted of erythromycin contents measured in milligrams, the SD is also in milligrams.

⚐ The Standard Deviation (SD)

The general purpose indicator of variability (dispersion).

It is often easier to comprehend the degree of variability in a set of data if we express it in relative terms. A typical example of this is when we want to express the precision of an analytical method.

The precision of an HPLC analysis for blood imipramine levels expressed as the coefficient of variation   An HPLC method for the measurement of blood levels of the antidepressant drug imipramine has been developed and as part of its validation we want to determine the reproducibility of its results. So, we analyse aliquots of the same blood sample on eight separate occasions. The mean result is 153 ± 9.33 ng/ml (±SD). The figure of ±9.33 ng/ml is our measure of assay variability. However, in isolation, this figure tells us precious little. To judge whether the method is acceptably precise we need to express the variability in a way that relates it to the amount being measured. The obvious way is as a percentage. The imprecision in the method is:

$$\pm 9.33/153 \times 100\% = \pm 6.1\%$$

We can now see that, for most purposes, the method would be acceptably precise. What we have just calculated is referred to as the coefficient of variation (CoV).

🔑 The coefficient of variation

$$\text{Coefficient of variation} = \frac{\text{SD}}{\text{mean}}$$

Expresses variation relative to the magnitude of the data.

The result could have been expressed as either a fraction (0.061) or a percentage (6.1 per cent). Because the coefficient of variation is a ratio, it is unitless (unlike the SD).

2.4 Quartiles – another way to describe data

The only real alternative to the mean and SD as descriptors for sets of measurements is the system of 'quartiles'. This enjoys a certain vogue in some research areas, but there are others where you will almost never see it used. We have already seen that the median is a value chosen to cut a set of data into two equal sized groups. Quartiles are an extension of that idea. Three quartiles are chosen so as to cut a data set into four equal-sized groups.

2.4.1 Quartiles – drug half-lives

The elimination half-lives of two synthetic steroids have been determined using two groups, each containing 15 volunteers. The results are shown in Table 2.5, with the values ranked from lowest to highest for each steroid.

Look at steroid number 1 first. Among the ranked half-lives, we highlight the half-lives that are ranked as fourth, eighth and twelfth and these will provide the three quartile values. We have now chopped the set of data into four equal-sized groups. There are three half-lives shorter than Q1, three between Q1 and Q2, three between Q2 and Q3 and three above Q3. We then check back for the actual values of the three highlighted cases and they are found to be:

$$Q1 = 5.4\,\text{h}$$
$$Q2 = 7.8\,\text{h}$$
$$Q3 = 10.0\,\text{h}$$

A similar exercise for steroid 2 yields quartiles values of 5.5, 6.6 and 7.8 h. The quartiles are indicated in Figure 2.7.

Table 2.5 Ranked half-lives for two steroids

Steroid 1		Steroid 2		
Rank	Half-life (h)	Rank	Half-life (h)	
1	3.9	1	4.4	
2	4.0	2	4.5	
4	**5.4**	4	**5.5** ←	4th ranked values = Q1
5	6.4	5	5.8	
6	6.5	6	5.9	
7	7.2	7	6.1	
8	**7.8**	8	**6.6** ←	8th ranked values = Q2 (Median)
9	8.6	9	7.2	
10	9.2	10	7.2	
11	9.3	11	7.3	
12	**10.0**	12	**7.8** ←	12th ranked values = Q3
13	10.6	13	8.5	
14	11.1	14	8.6	
15	15.8	15	9.1	

The second quartile (median) as an indicator of central tendency The second quartile has half the observations above it and half below and is therefore synonymous with the median. We have already established that the median is a useful and robust indicator of central tendency, especially when there are some extreme

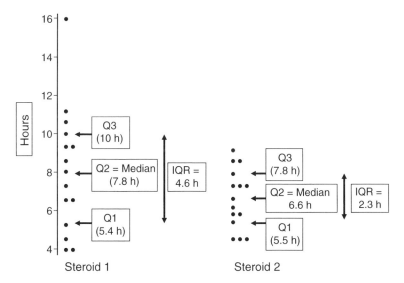

Figure 2.7 Steroid half-lives. The median (second quartile) indicates generally longer elimination half-lives for steroid 1 relative to steroid 2. The interquartile range indicates greater variability for the first steroid

outlying values.

$$Q2 \text{ or median} = 7.8\,\text{h for first steroid and } 6.6\,\text{h for the second.}$$

The median values suggest that somewhat longer half-lives are seen with the first steroid.

The inter-quartile range as an indicator of dispersion   The inter-quartile range is defined as the difference between the upper and lower quartiles (Q3 – Q1). So, for steroid 1:

$$\text{Inter-quartile range} = 10.0 - 5.4 = 4.6\,\text{h}$$

The fact that the interquartile-range does reflect dispersion can be appreciated if you compare steroid 1 with number 2. With steroid 2 the half-lives are visibly less disperse and quartiles 1 and 3 are closer together. In this case:

$$\text{Inter-quartile range} = 7.8 - 5.5 = 2.3\,\text{h}$$

The inter-quartile range for the half life of steroid 2 is thus only half that for steroid 1, duly reflecting its less variable nature.

Just as the median is a robust indicator of central tendency, the interquartile range is a robust indicator of dispersion. Take the longest half-life seen with steroid 1 (15.8 h) and consider what would have happened if that individual had produced a half-life of 100 h (or any other extreme value). The answer is that it would make absolutely no difference to the inter-quartile range. The value of 15.8 h is already something of an outlier, but it had no undue effect on the inter-quartile range.

The standard deviation is much less robust. If there was an odd individual with an extremely long half-life for either steroid, then its value would deviate massively from the group mean and the SD would be inflated.

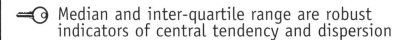 Median and inter-quartile range are robust indicators of central tendency and dispersion

The second quartile (median) and inter-quartile range can be used as an alternative method for describing the central tendency and dispersion of a set of measured data. Both are robust and can be useful where there are occasional extreme values.

2.4.2   Other quantiles

Having met the median and quartiles, which divide sets of data into two or four ranges, we can then extend the principle to any system where $n - 1$ points are chosen to divide our data into n ranges. These methods are collectively referred to as 'quantile' systems. Thus, the median and quartiles are specific examples of quantiles. Quantile systems that cut data into more than four ranges are really only useful where there are large numbers of observations.

The only other quantile systems that are used with any regularity are quintiles, deciles and centiles. There are four quintiles, which divide data into five ranges, nine deciles for 10 ranges and 99 centiles that produce 100 ranges. The ninth decile is thus equivalent to the ninetieth centile and both indicate a point that ranks 10 per cent from the top of a set of values.

A classic use of quartiles arose in the UK as part of the settlement of a long and bitter strike over pay in the fire service. A long-term solution was arrived at whereby fire personnel's pay would be set at 'The upper quartile of industrial wages'. This meant that pay would be set at such a level that fire personnel would receive higher levels of pay than three-quarters of industrial workers, but less then the wealthiest 25 per cent. (It also led to an unusually high level of understanding of quantile systems among firemen!)

⚼ Quantile systems

Quantile systems divide ranked data sets into groups with equal numbers of observations in each group. Specifically:

3 *quartiles* divide data into four equal-sized groups;
4 *quintiles* divide data five ways;
9 *deciles* divide it 10 ways;
99 *centiles* divide it 100 ways.

2.5 Using computer packages to generate descriptive statistics

2.5.1 Excel

The one thing at which Excel does not excel is statistical analysis. The (very basic) level of material covered in this chapter is about at (if not beyond) the limit of its capabilities. It can be used to generate means, medians, SDs and quartiles, but while the first three are OK, the quartile values generated are somewhat unconventional and will not be pursued further. The mean, median and SD of a data set can be generated by using either worksheet functions or the Data Analysis tool.

To use worksheet functions, enter the tablet erythromycin contents from Table 2.4 into the first two columns of an Excel spread-sheet (assume titles in A1 and B1 and the two sets of data in A2 : A11 and B2 : B11), and then enter the following formulae into A12 : A14 and B12 : B14:

$$A12 = \text{Average}(A2 : A11)$$
$$A13 = \text{StDev}(A2 : A11)$$
$$A14 = \text{Median}(A2 : A11)$$
$$B12 = \text{Average}(B2 : B11)$$
$$B13 = (\text{StDev}(B2 : B11)$$
$$B14 = \text{Median}(B2 : B11)$$

(Notice that the formulae must be preceded by an equals sign, as shown.)

The appropriate means, medians and standard deviations will be displayed. (You might also want to try setting up a spread-sheet to perform the full calculations for the SD as shown in Table 2.4, just to reinforce exactly how this is derived.)

To use the Data Analysis tool, enter the data as above and then proceed through the menus Tools then Data Analysis, then select Descriptive Statistics. In the box labelled 'Input Range', enter A2:B11 and tick the box for 'Summary statistics'. The mean, median and standard deviation will be shown for both data sets, but you will probably need to widen the columns to make the output clear.

When you open the Tools menu, Data Analysis may not appear on the menu, in which case it needs to be installed. To do this, go back to the Tools menu and select Add-Ins . . . and tick the box for Analysis ToolPak.

2.5.2 Other statistical packages

General approach in this book   The web site associated with this book gives detailed instructions for generating means, medians, standard deviations and quartiles using Minitab and SPSS. (Instructions for other packages will be added as and when time permits. Check web site for latest features.)

For all statistical procedures, the book will provide general instructions that will certainly be appropriate for SPSS and Minitab, but also for most other packages. These will cover those aspects that are fairly standard:

- the pattern in which data should be entered;

- the information that will need to be entered in order to run the routine;

- what information to look for in the output.

The one thing that is completely variable between packages is navigation through menu structures to trigger a particular routine, so this is not covered here.

To illustrate what to look for, generic output is provided. This is not formatted in the same manner as that from any specific package, but contains details that all packages ought to generate.

Table 2.6 Generic output of descriptive statistics for the erythromycin data shown in Table 2.4

Descriptive statistics: erythro

	n	Mean	SD	SEM	Median	Q1	Q3
Alpha	10	248.7	8.72	2.76	249.00	241.50	255.50
Bravo	10	251.1	3.78	1.20	251.00	249.25	254.25

Obtaining descriptive statistics for the erythromycin data   The data are generally entered into a column (or into separate columns if several data sets are to be described). Once the menu structure has been navigated to select the Descriptive Statistics routine, the only additional information to be supplied is which column(s) contain the relevant data. Table 2.6 shows generic output.

The number of observations (n) and the statistics referred to in this chapter should be fairly obvious. The second quartile (Q2) is generally not shown as it is the same as the median. The SEM may not be familiar at the moment, but is an important statistic that will be described in Chapter 4.

2.6 Chapter summary

When choosing a descriptive statistic we need to be aware of whether the data contains extreme outlying values and whether it forms a single cluster (unimodal) or several (polymodal). We should also think about what use is intended for the statistic we quote.

The mean, median and mode are all indicators of central tendency and tell us about the magnitude of the figures within our data.

- The mean is synonymous with the average.

- The median is the middle ranking value.

- The mode (or modes) is/are the most frequently occurring value either overall or within each cluster of values.

For most purposes there is a pecking order with the mean being most useful and therefore the prime candidate, then the median and finally the mode (or modes) only used in desperation. So long as the data are unimodal and not unduly affected by extreme values, the mean is the obvious choice. Where the data are badly affected by outliers, the median may provide a better impression of a typical value. Only the modes can properly describe polymodal data.

The standard deviation is an indicator of dispersion. It tells us about the variability among the figures within our data. The coefficient of variation describes relative variability by expressing the SD as a ratio to the mean.

The three quartile values indicate the figures that appear 25, 50 and 75 per cent of the way up the list of data when it has been ranked. The second quartile is synonymous with the median and can act as an indicator of central tendency. The interquartile range (difference between first and third quartile) is an indicator of dispersion. The median and interquartile range are 'robust' statistics, which means that they are more resistant to the effects of occasional extreme values than the mean and SD. The robustness of the median can be abused to hide the existence of aberrant data.

Detailed instructions are provided for the calculation of the mean, median and SD (but not quartiles) using Microsoft Excel. Readers are referred to the accompanying web site for detailed instructions on generating all these descriptive statistics (including quartiles) using Minitab or SPSS. Generalized instructions that should be relevant to most statistical packages are provided in the book.

3
The normal distribution

This chapter will . . .

- Describe the normal distribution

- Suggest visual methods for detecting data that do not follow a normal distribution

- Describe the proportion of individual values that should fall within specified ranges

3.1 What is a normal distribution?

Many of the things we measure show a characteristic distribution, with the bulk of individuals clustered around the group mean and then cases become steadily rarer as we move further away from the mean.

In the previous chapter, Figure 2.5 showed a sample of 500 tablets from an 'Alpha' tabletting machine. The bulk of the tablets were clustered in the central region with between 240 and 260 mg erythromycin. Out at the extremes (less than 230 or more than 270 mg), cases were very rare. Five hundred is quite a large sample and yet the histogram was still a long way from a perfectly smooth shape. With larger and larger samples we would gradually move towards a graph that followed the superimposed curve. The idealized curve in Figure 2.5 is what is referred to as a normal distribution. It looks like a cross section through a bell.

Essential Statistics for the Pharmaceutical Sciences   Philip Rowe
© 2007 John Wiley & Sons, Ltd   ISBN 9780 470 03470 5 (HB)   ISBN 9780 470 03468 2 (PB)

When a curve is superimposed on the data from the Bravo machine (Figure 2.6), it has different proportions (taller and narrower) because these tablets are less variable and cluster more tightly around the mean. However, both sets of data follow normal distributions.

⚬ Normal distributions can vary in appearance

Normal distributions may be squat and broad if there is a large SD, or tall and thin with a small SD.

3.2 Identifying data that are not normally distributed

3.2.1 Does it matter?

Many of the statistical techniques that we are going to look at in later chapters only work properly if the data being analysed follow a normal distribution. The requirement is more than just a statistical nicety. In some cases, we can get quite ludicrous results by applying methods that assume normality to severely non-normal data. An unfortunate side-effect of the very term 'normal' distribution is a subliminal suggestion that such distributions are what we would normally expect to obtain and anything else is, in some way, abnormal. That sadly is not the case.

3.2.2 How to spot non-normal data

There are a number of statistical tests that will allegedly help in deciding whether data deviate from a normal distribution. However, in the author's experience the results of such tests tend to be difficult to interpret in real-life situations. What I am going to suggest is a simple visual inspection of histograms of data, and I have highlighted specific features that indicate non-normality.

There are three visual characteristics that any true normal distribution will possess. Strictly speaking, possession of all three of these does not guarantee normality, but it is rare to find data sets that fit all three criteria and still manage to be sufficiently non-normal to cause serious practical difficulties. The three characteristics are:

- The data are unimodal.

- The distribution is symmetrical.

- The frequencies decline steadily as we move towards higher or lower values, without any sudden, sharp cut-off.

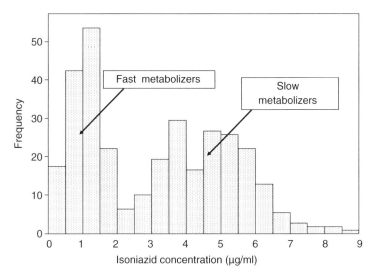

Figure 3.1 Bimodal data. Isoniazid concentrations (µg/ml) 6 h after a standard oral dose

By way of illustration, the three cases below show infractions of each of the criteria in turn. You do need to be aware that, unless samples are very large, histograms will not exactly follow the classical, pleasing-to-the-eye bell curve. What you need to check for are obvious and gross deviations from a normal distribution.

Data with a polymodal distribution   If we give a series of patients a standard oral dose of the anti-tuberculosis drug isoniazid, obtain a blood sample from each individual 6 h later and determine the isoniazid concentrations of those samples, the results will probably look like Figure 3.1. The data are bimodal, because the metabolism of isoniazid is genetically controlled and we all fall into one of two groups – fast or slow metabolizers. The fast metabolizers form the cluster at the low end of the concentration scale and the slow metabolizers form a distinct group with higher levels.

  Any attempt to apply statistical methods that rely upon a normal distribution to data like this is likely to end in nonsensical conclusions.

Data that are severely skewed   A candidate anti-cancer drug is being extracted from plant leaves. Examples of the plant have been obtained from a wide range of geographical regions and each plant has been analysed for its content of the drug. Figure 3.2 shows the results. The pattern is far from symmetrical. Instead we have a long tail of results on one side, not balanced on the other. This is referred to as a 'skewed' distribution. Again, any attempt to analyse such data using statistical methods that assume a normal distribution is likely to lead to very real practical difficulties.

  The skewing seen in Figure 3.2 is referred to as 'positive skew', because the long tail extends towards high values. It is also possible to encounter negative skew. Figure 3.3 shows generalized examples of both types of skew.

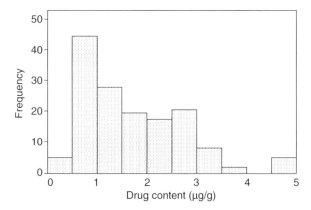

Figure 3.2   Skewed data. Drug content (milligrams per gram of dried plant tissue) of a series of individual plants

Skew often arises when results are constrained in one direction, but not the other. The drug concentrations for example (Figure 3.2) cannot be less than zero, but can extend virtually without limit to the right. Practical experience suggests that positive skew is quite common in data from biological and medical research – negative skew less so. This is largely because many endpoints cannot fall below zero, but it is rarer for values to push up against an upper limit.

Data that are sharply truncated above and/or below the mean   Patients report the amount of disability they are suffering as a result of gout. A 'visual analogue scale' is used to gather the information. A scale is printed with labels along its length reading 'minimal disability', 'moderate disability' and 'severe disability'. Patients make a mark on the scale at a point that they feel describes their situation. The scale is then divided into eight equal lengths and each patient's mark on the scale converted to a score of 1–8, with 8 being the greatest degree of disability. The final result is an ordinal scale of measurement. A histogram of the scores is shown in Figure 3.4.

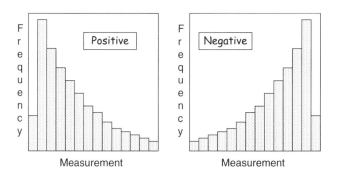

Figure 3.3   Positive and negative skew

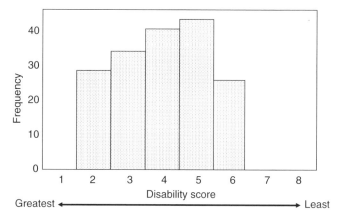

Figure 3.4 Data with sudden cut-offs. Patients' self-assessment score for degree of disability due to gout

For whatever reason, the patients have only used a limited, central part of the available scale. No patient has considered their condition to be at either extreme. For this to be a proper normal distribution, there should be gradual declines in frequencies below 2 and above 6. Instead we see these sudden, sharp cut-offs.

Ordered scores on scales with a limited number of possible values are notorious for producing patterns that are wildly non-normal and we tend to avoid analysing such data using methods where a normal distribution is a pre-requisite.

⚷ Identifying data that is not normally distributed

With many statistical routines, we must avoid data sets that are markedly non-normally distributed. If data has all of the characteristics below, it is unlikely to be so non-normal as to cause any practical problems:

- unimodal;

- symmetrical;

- no sharp cut-offs at high or low values.

3.3 Proportions of individuals within one or two standard deviations of the mean

Because the shape of the normal distribution is exactly mathematically defined, a predictable proportion of individuals falls within any given distance of the mean.

3.3.1 Approximately two-thirds lie within 1 SD of the mean

For example, assume that, in a large group of subjects, the mean clearance of a drug is 10 l/h with a standard deviation of 1.5 l/h. We can then define a range of clearances that fall within 1 SD of the mean. One standard deviation below the mean is 8.5 l/h and 1 SD above is 11.5 l/h.

It is a general property of normally distributed data that 68 per cent of individuals fall within 1 SD of the mean. So, assuming that the clearance data follow a true normal distribution, 68 per cent of individuals should fall within the range calculated above. With 68 per cent in this central range, the remaining 32 per cent must constitute the two tails of individuals with relatively high or low clearances. Because the normal distribution is symmetrical, this 32 per cent is distributed as 16 per cent in each of the two tails. This is shown in Figure 3.5. The proportion 68 per cent may not seem particularly memorable, but if you think of it as near enough two-thirds of individuals falling within 1 SD of the mean, it is more likely to stick.

3.3.2 Approximately 95 per cent lie within 2 SDs of the mean

It is then possible to extend this principal and calculate the proportion of individuals who fall within any given number of SDs of the mean. In standard tables, you can look up how many people should fall within 1, 2, 3, 1½ or any other number of SDs of the mean. However, the only other case of special interest is that approximately 95 per cent of individuals fall within the range ±2 SDs from the mean. Taking our clearance values, 2 SDs (3 l/h) below the mean would be 7.0 l/h and 2 above would be 13.0 l/h. Figure 3.6 shows the 95 per cent of individuals who fall in the wider range between ±2

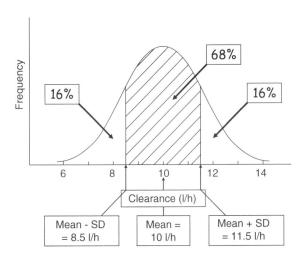

Figure 3.5 Approximately two-thirds of individuals with a drug clearance within 1 SD of the mean. (mean 10.0 ± 1.5 l/h)

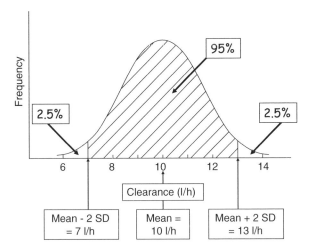

Figure 3.6 Approximatelt 95 per cent of individuals with a drug clearance within 2 SDs of the mean. (mean 10.0 ± 1.5 l/h); this is often quoted as the 'normal range'

SDs. The remaining (approximately 5 per cent) of individuals are then found in the two small, extreme tails.

Proportions of individuals within given ranges

For data that follows a normal distribution:

• about two-thirds of individuals will have values within 1 SD of the mean;

• about 95 per cent of individuals will have values within 2 SD of the mean.

3.3.3 'Normal range'

For practical purposes people frequently find it convenient to identify a 'normal range' for a particular parameter. For example, clinically, we may measure all sorts of ions and enzymes in a patient's blood and then we want to be able to spot any abnormal values that may be of importance in diagnosis and treatment. To make it easier to spot these interesting values, clinicians like to establish a 'normal range' for each substance measured. Then, all they have to do is check for values outside the official normal range.

However, if the parameter is normally distributed in ordinary healthy people, then there is no nice clear cut point at which the values become suddenly 'abnormal'. There will be perfectly healthy people with values out in the tails of the distribution. A common approach is an arbitrary declaration that the middle 95 per cent of values are 'normal'. A normal range can then be arrived at by taking the mean ± 2 SDs. Assuming the parameter to be normally distributed, this will then include about 95 per cent of individuals.

The problem of course, is that the remaining 5 per cent, who may be perfectly healthy, are suddenly condemned as 'abnormal'. It is very easy to condemn such a system as arbitrary; however, in many cases there is no better system available and it is difficult to proceed without agreeing some sort of normal range.

⊶ 'Normal ranges'

Normal ranges are frequently based on the mean ± 2 SDs. These need to be treated with some scepticism, but are often the only pragmatic approach available.

3.4 Chapter summary

Data that follow a normal distribution are clustered around the mean, with declining frequencies as we move to values further away. A graph of these frequencies looks like a cross-section through a bell. It is symmetrical.

The shape depends upon the variability within the data. With a low SD, the data are all clustered tightly around the mean and the distribution is tall and thin. With more scattered data (higher SD), the distribution is low and wide.

Many statistical routines are liable to produce misleading results if applied to data that depart severely from a normal distribution. It is recommended that a check for gross non-normality should be made by producing a histogram of the data and checking that the distibution is unimodal, symmetrical and free from sharp cut-offs at either high or low values.

Data that are not symmetrical are described as 'skewed'. In positive skew, there are outlying extreme values, all (or most) of which are above the mean. In negative skew, the outliers are below the mean. Positive skew is quite common in biological and medical data.

In a normally distributed data set, about two-thirds of individual values will lie within 1 SD of the mean and about 95 per cent within 2 SD. The 'normal range' for a value is frequently equated with the range mean $\pm$ 2SD. This is pragmatically useful, but the 5 per cent of values outside this range can be overly simplistically interpreted as evidence that the individuals concerned are 'abnormal'.

4

Sampling from populations – the SEM

This chapter will ...

- Distinguish between samples and populations

- Describe the way in which sample size and the SD jointly influence random sampling error

- Show how the standard error of the mean (SEM) can be used to indicate the likely extent of random sampling error

---

4.1 Samples and populations

Statisticians carry on endlessly about two particular terms – 'population' and 'sample'. There is in fact good reason for the emphasis placed on these concepts and we need to be clear about the distinction.

4.1.1. Population

One of the hall-marks of good research is that there should be a clear definition of the target group of individuals (or objects) about whom we are aiming to draw a conclusion. The term 'population' is used to cover all the individuals who fall within

Essential Statistics for the Pharmaceutical Sciences   Philip Rowe
© 2007 John Wiley & Sons, Ltd   ISBN 9780 470 03470 5 (HB)   ISBN 9780 470 03468 2 (PB)

that target group. The experimenter can define the target group as widely or narrowly as they see fit. Some experiments may be very general, with the intention that our conclusions should be applicable to the entire human race or all the cats or all the dogs on the planet. In other cases, the target may be much more narrowly defined, perhaps all the females aged 55–65 with moderate to severe rheumatoid-arthritis, living in North America. The size of the population will vary accordingly. At one extreme (all humans) there might be 6000 million of them, whereas the group with arthritis (defined above) might contain only a few million.

⌐O Population

The complete collection of individuals about whom we wish to draw some conclusion.

While the sizes of populations may vary, they all tend to be too large for us to be able to study them in their entirety. Of course, it is possible to define a population so tightly that the numbers become manageable. Left-handed, red-headed, males aged 95–100, living in Inverness, Scotland might well constitute a population small enough for us to be able to study all its members. However, with all due respect to these sinistral, Scottish red-heads, it is unlikely that anybody would be very interested in such a narrowly constituted group. As a general rule, any population that is worth studying will be too large to study.

4.1.2 Sample

Since it is usually impossible to study a whole population, real science is carried out on smaller samples randomly selected from the larger population. The sample is unlikely to be of any direct interest to the reader. However, it is of indirect interest – the hope is that we can use the sample as a tool to throw light on the nature of the general population.

⌐O Sample

A random selection of individuals from the population we wish to study.

4.2 From sample to population

However, there must be some doubts about the validity of using data that relate to one thing (a sample) to draw conclusions about something else (the population). Is

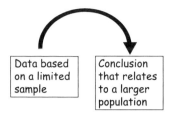

Figure 4.1 The great leap of faith required when drawing a conclusion about a population, based only on limited data from a smaller sample

this leap from sample to population justified? As Figure 4.1 implies, we need to maintain a healthy scepticism about such extrapolations.

If our sample is in fact not representative of the underlying population, then instead of throwing light on the situation, it will positively mislead us. So, we will next consider the various and nefarious ways in which a sample might misrepresent the population.

🔑 From sample to population

The purpose of a sample is to estimate properties of the broader population, such as its mean value, but we need to be alert to the possibility that a sample may misrepresent the population.

4.3 Types of sampling error

There are two distinct types of error that may arise – bias and random error.

4.3.1 Bias – systematic error

It is all too easy to take samples, which are virtually guaranteed to produce an average value that is predictably above (or predictably below) the true population mean. In some cases the problem is blindingly obvious and in others more subtle. A couple of examples follow:

- If we want to determine average alcohol consumption among the citizens of a given city, we might recruit our subjects by giving out questionnaires in a bar in the town centre. The average figure at which we would arrive is pretty obviously going to be higher than the true average for all citizens of the city – very few of the town's teetotallers will be present in the bar.

- A drug causes raised blood pressure as a side-effect in some users and we want to see how large this effect is. We might recruit patients who have been using the drug for a year and measure their blood pressures. In this case the bias is less blindingly obvious, but equally inevitable. We will almost certainly understate the hypertensive effect of the drug as all the most severely affected patients will have been forced to withdraw from using the drug. We will be left with a select group who are relatively unaffected.

⚏◯ Bias or systematic error

A consistent form of mis-estimation of the mean. Either most such samples would over-estimate the value or most would under-estimate it.

The principal characteristics of bias are

1. If we were to repeat the same sampling procedure several times, we could pretty much guarantee that we would make an error in the same direction every time. With the drink survey, we would always tend to over-estimate consumption and, with the hypertension study, we would consistently under-estimate the side effect.

2. Bias arises from flaws in our experimental design.

3. We can remove the bias by improving our experimental design (always assuming that we recognize the error of our ways!).

4.3.2 Random error

Now take an essentially sound experimental design. We want to determine the average elimination half-life of a new anti-diabetic drug in type II diabetics aged 50–75, within Western Europe. We recruit several hospitals scattered throughout Western Europe and they draw up a census of all the appropriately aged, type II diabetics under their care. From these lists we then randomly select potential subjects.

Although this design is unlikely to produce a biased estimate, it is still very unlikely that our sample will produce a mean half-life that exactly matches the true mean value for the whole population. All samples contain some individuals that have above-average values but their effect is more-or-less cancelled out by others with low values. However, the devil is in that expression 'more-or-less'. In our experiment on half-lives, it would be remarkable if the individuals with shorter than average half-lives exactly counterbalanced the effect of those with relatively long half-lives. Most real samples will have some residual over- or under-estimation.

However, what we have just described is random error, and there is an important difference from bias. There is no longer any way that we could predict whether error would take the form of over- or under-estimation. Indeed, if we carried out such a survey repeatedly, we would probably suffer very similar numbers of over- and under-estimates.

 Random error

Any given sample has an equal chance of under- or over-estimating the population mean value.

The characteristics of random error are:

1. Over- and under-estimation are equally likely.

2. Even the best designed experiments are subject to random error.

3. It is impossible get rid of random error.

4.3.3 The rest of this book is concerned with random error only – not bias

For the rest of this book we will be concerned solely with the problem of random error. Bias just should not be there – good experimental design should see it off. However, random error is ever with us and the science of statistics is there to allow us to draw conclusions despite its presence. Statistics will not make random error disappear, it just allows us to live with it.

 Life's certainties

In this world, nothing is certain but death, taxes and random sampling error. (Modified from Benjamin Franklin's original.)

4.4 What factors control the extent of random sampling error?

To illustrate the points made in this section we will refer back to the two tabletting machines introduced in Section 2.3. One machine (Alpha) produced more variable tablets than the other (Bravo). We will assume that the long-term average drug content of the tablets corresponds to their nominal content of 250 mg.

Two factors control the extent of random sampling error. One is almost universally recognized, but the other is less widely appreciated.

4.4.1 Sample size

If we take random samples of tablets made on an Alpha machine, the accuracy of the sample means will depend on how well any high and low values happen to cancel out. Two samples are shown in Table 4.1.

We know from Figure 2.5 that the true population mean for erythromycin content is very close to the nominal figure of 250 mg. In both samples an odd outlying high value (marked **) has crept in. Because the first sample is small, the outlier has displaced the sample mean considerably above the true population mean. There is also an odd value in the second sample, but it is now only one observation among 12, and so the sample mean remains much closer to the true value.

Most of us recognize that, the larger a sample is, the more likely it is to reflect the true underlying situation. However, it does not matter how big a sample is, we must always anticipate some random sampling error.

There is a constant tension between the statistician who wants the most precise (i.e. largest) possible samples and the experimenter who wants to keep the experiment as quick and cheap (i.e. small) as possible. Real-world experimental design always ends up as a compromise between these conflicting priorities.

Table 4.1 Erythromycin contents (mg) for two random samples of tablets (both from an Alpha machine)

	Sample 1 ($n = 3$)	Sample 2 ($n = 12$)
	246	258
	253	249
	270**	258
		249
		270**
		253
		237
		246
		259
		248
		242
		258
Mean	256.33	252.25

🗝️ Sample size (statistician's point of view)

Big samples: good.
Small samples: bad.

4.4.2 Variability within the data

The second factor that influences random error is more easily overlooked. Table 4.2 shows a typical result, if we take two random samples of tablets – one for an Alpha and the other for a Bravo machine. The secret is to remember that the tablets from the Alpha machine are more variable than the Bravo ones.

Because the tablets produced by the Alpha machine are so variable, an outlying value can be high or low enough to do quite a lot of damage. In the sample from the Alpha machine there happens to be some very low values (e.g. 235 and 240 mg). Consequently our sample mean for this machine differs rather badly from the true population mean (At 247.33 mg it is 2.67 mg below the assumed true population mean of 250 mg). However, extreme values are rarer among tablets produced by the more consistent Bravo machine and so it is no surprise that the sample is not spoiled by any similar cluster of high or low values. As a result, the sample mean for this machine remains closer to the true population mean. (At 248.92 mg, it is only 1.08 mg below the ideal figure.)

Table 4.2 Erythromycin contents (mg) for two random samples of tablets (one from an Alpha and the other from a Bravo machine)

	Alpha	Bravo
	252	254
	240	246
	243	247
	243	251
	250	254
	242	247
	257	251
	253	250
	251	242
	246	250
	235	247
	256	248
Mean $\pm$ SD	247.33 $\pm$ 6.85	248.92 $\pm$ 3.45

Therefore, the other general rule is that samples means based on highly variable data are themselves rather variable and may provide a poor reflection of the true situation. With non-varying data, almost all samples will be pretty accurate.

⚷ Variability in the data (everybody's point of view)

Big SDs: bad.
Small SDs: good.

Unlike sample size, the SD is not primarily under the control of the experimenter. Tablets from the Alpha machine simply are rather variable and there is very little we can do about it. (Although, the directors of the Alpha Corporation probably should.) About the only thing we can do is to make sure that we do not increase the variability within our data by adding unnecessary measurement error. If we use imprecise measurement techniques, the final SD among the data we collect will be even greater than the intrinsic variability of the parameter in question. In this particular case, it is bad enough that the tablets are so variable, but if we then use an imprecise analytical technique, the figures will end up being even more scattered.

4.5 Estimating likely sampling error – the SEM

We have identified the two relevant factors:

- sample size;

- standard deviation within the data.

We are now in a position to estimate likely sampling error for any given experimental situation.

At one extreme, if we take a small sample from a population of highly varying data, we must accept that our sample mean may be wildly misleading. In contrast, a large sample from non-varying data will produce a sample mean that is virtually guaranteed to be very close to the true population mean.

4.5.1 SEM

Frustratingly, we cannot calculate exactly how much sampling error will be present in any individual sample. The error is random in nature and with any given sample we may over or underestimate the true situation, or (if it was an unusually lucky sample) we might be almost bang on. What we can estimate is a typical amount of sampling error that would occur with a given sampling regime. This is referred to as the standard error of the mean (SEM). The purpose of the SEM is to provide an estimate of the likely sampling error that should be anticipated, given the size of the sample and the variability among the data being sampled.

🔑 **Standard error of the mean (SEM)**

Estimate of the likely extent of sampling error, based upon the sample size and the SD among the data being sampled.

4.5.2 The technical definition of SEM

For practical purposes, the only essential thing to understand is that the SEM is a indicator of likely sampling error. This short section offers a technical definition of the SEM. If you do not follow it, no matter. It is the purpose of the SEM that is crucial.

A common approach in statistics is to ask 'What would happen if we were to repeat a sampling procedure many times?' In this case, the question we ask is 'What would happen if we were to take repeated samples and calculate the mean of each sample?' Fortunately, we do not actually have to take real repeated samples. We can calculate what would happen if we did, based on the fact that we know sampling error is dependent upon sample size and SD. An example of hypothetical repeated re-sampling is shown in Figure 4.2. Note that the horizontal axis represents the mean values of samples, not the individual values that go into the samples. The sample means mainly cluster around the true population mean, but there are a few outlying results badly above and below. These sample means themselves form a normal

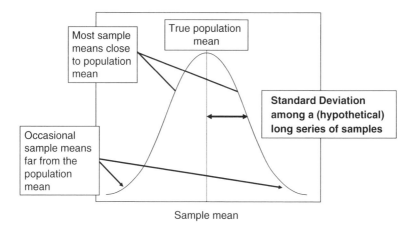

Figure 4.2 The SEM is the SD among hypothetical repeated sample means

distribution. We can indicate the variability among these sample estimates in the usual way – we quote their SD. This SD among a large number of hypothetical sample means is then given the special name of the standard error of the mean.

🔑 Definition of the SEM

The SD among (hypothetical) repeated sample means from the same population.

4.5.3 The SEM in action

The SEM is shown in action in Figure 4.3. This contrasts what would happen if we were to take either small or large samples from the same population. Small samples are not very precise and the sample means would be badly spread out. Hence, the SEM would be large. With the larger samples, the means would be more tightly clustered and the SEM smaller. The SEM has thus achieved what we wanted. It has acted as a indicator of likely sampling error – large errors are quite likely with the smaller samples, but big samples are less error prone.

We could construct a diagram similar to Figure 4.3, to compare the situation with small and large SDs. In that case, the spread of sample means (and hence the SEM) would be greatest when there was a large SD.

4.5.4 Calculation of the SEM

The calculation of the SEM is based upon the SD and the sample size, as shown in Figure 4.4. The form of the diagram used in Figure 4.4 will be used throughout this

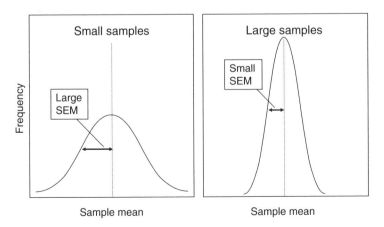

Figure 4.3   The SEM in action – small and large samples

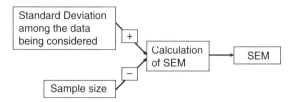

Figure 4.4   Calculation of the standard error of the mean. Signs indicate whether increases in a factor would increase (+) or decrease (−) the SEM

book. The idea is to avoid equations, while still identifying the factors that influence a particular outcome and also indicating the direction of their influence. Thus, Figure 4.4 tells us that the factors governing the SEM are the SD and the sample size, then the plus sign indicates that the SD is positively related to the SEM. In other words the greater the SD, the greater the SEM will be. The minus sign indicates a negative relationship – the greater the sample size, the lower the SEM will be.

In this particular case the mathematical equation underlying the block diagram is so simple that we could have used it without causing excessive consternation to even the less numerate:

$$\text{SEM} = \frac{\text{SD}}{\sqrt{n}}$$

$\sqrt{n}$ being the square-root of the sample size.

While the actual equation is reasonably digestible in this case, many of the other relationships we will be looking at are far more complex and the block diagrams are much more accessible. In fact, we do not need to worry about even this equation, as stats packages invariably report the SEM as part of their descriptive statistics routines (see Table 2.6).

4.5.5 Obtaining SEMs for the samples of erythromycin contents in Tables 4.1 and 4.2

It would be no great hardship to calculate the SEMs manually, as below.

For Table 4.1:

For $n = 3$: SEM $= 12.34/\sqrt{3}$ For $n = 12$: SEM $= 8.93/\sqrt{12}$
$\quad\quad\quad\quad = 12.34/1.73$ $\quad\quad\quad\quad\quad = 8.93/3.46$
$\quad\quad\quad\quad = 7.13$ mg $\quad\quad\quad\quad\quad = 2.58$ mg

For Table 4.2 ($n = 12$):

Alpha SEM $= 6.85/\sqrt{12}$ Bravo SEM $= 3.45/\sqrt{12}$
$\quad\quad\quad\quad = 6.85/3.46$ $\quad\quad\quad\quad\quad = 3.45/3.46$
$\quad\quad\quad\quad = 1.98$ mg $\quad\quad\quad\quad\quad = 0.996$ mg

However, computers are quicker (and more reliable). Excel does not offer the SEM as a standard worksheet function, but it is included in the output from the Data Analysis tool (see Chapter 2). Both Minitab and SPSS include it in their Descriptive Statistics routines.

For Table 4.1, the first sample contained only three observations and is therefore thoroughly unreliable. Its SEM is given as 7.13 mg. The second sample's SEM is considerably smaller (2.58 mg), reflecting its greater size and reliability.

For Table 4.2, the SEM for Alpha is 1.98 mg and for Bravo only 0.996 mg. The sample of tablets from the Alpha machine is liable to be distorted by somewhat outlying values and so the SEM is relatively high. In contrast, the mean based on the tablets from the Bravo machine will be more reliable as it is less likely to contain badly outlying values and the SEM is correspondingly lower.

4.6 Offsetting sample size against standard deviation

Because sample quality is adversely affected when the standard deviation is large, it is difficult to work with such data. However, it is not impossible. Figure 4.4 shows us that the SEM can be controlled to any required value by adjusting the sample size. Even if the data are very variable, a suitably low SEM can be achieved by increasing the sample size. In contrast, with data of low variability, it is possible to enjoy the luxury of small sample sizes and still obtain a respectable SEM.

⚷ Offsetting SD and sample size

Sample sizes can be adjusted to restrict the SEM to any pre-selected value, by taking account of the size of the SD.

4.7 Chapter summary

Scientific data generally consist of randomly selected samples from larger populations. The purpose of the sample is to estimate the mean etc of the population.

A sample may mis-estimate the population mean as a result of bias or random sampling error. Bias is a predictable over- or under-estimation, arising from poor experimental design. Random error arises due to the unavoidable risk that any randomly selected sample may over-represent either low or high values.

The extent of random sampling error is governed by the sample size and the SD of the data. Small samples are subject to greater random error than large ones. Data with a high SD are subject to greater sampling error than that with low variability.

The standard error of the mean is used to indicate the extent of random sampling error that would typically arise with a particular sampling scheme. It is calculated by taking account of the sample size and the SD. The technical definition of the SEM is that it is the SD that would be found among a hypothetical long series of sample means drawn from the relevant population. Examples are given where the SEM is greater for a small sample than a large one, and also where it is greater for data with a high SD than where it is low.

5

Ninety-five per cent confidence interval for the mean

This chapter will . . .

- Describe the concept of a confidence interval (CI)

- Explain what is meant by '95 per cent confidence'

- Show how other levels of confidence could be used

- Show that the width of a confidence interval is dependent upon sample size and SD and the level of confidence required

- Describe one-sided CIs

- Describe the CI for the difference between two means

- Emphasize that data needs to adhere reasonably well to a normal distribution, if it is to be used to generate a 95 percent CI for the mean

- Show how data transformations may be used to convert data to a normal distribution

Essential Statistics for the Pharmaceutical Sciences Philip Rowe
© 2007 John Wiley & Sons, Ltd   ISBN 9780 470 03470 5 (HB)   ISBN 9780 470 03468 2 (PB)

5.1 What is a confidence interval?

We have already established that a mean derived from a sample is unlikely to be a perfect estimate of the population mean. Since it is not possible to produce a single reliable value, a commonly used way forward is to quote a range within which we are reasonably confident the true population mean lies. Such a range is referred to as a 'confidence interval'.

The mean derived from the sample remains the best available estimate of the population mean and is referred to as the 'point estimate'. We add and subtract a suitable amount to the point estimate to define upper and lower limits of an interval. We then state that the true population mean probably lies somewhere within the range we have now defined.

5.2 How wide should the interval be?

We will use some data where we have measured the quantity of imipramine (an antidepressant) in nominally 25 mg tablets. Nine tablets have been randomly selected from a large batch and found to contain the following amounts (See Table 5.1). We want to calculate a confidence interval for the mean.

The obvious question is how wide should the interval be? Clearly, the wider the interval is, the greater our confidence that it will include the true population mean. For example, interval (a) in Figure 5.1 only covers a range of about 0.2 mg. Since we know, from the SEM, that a sampling error of 0.3 mg is perfectly credible, we would have very little confidence that the true mean will fall within any such narrowly defined interval.

In contrast, interval (c) is so wide as to make it almost inconceivable that the population mean would not be included. While this high level of confidence is reassuring, the price we have paid is that the interval is now singularly unhelpful. The information that the mean probably falls within a range which covers all of the individual data points, is hardly novel.

Table 5.1 Imipramine content (mg) of nine randomly selected tablets

24.7
25.8
26.7
25.5
24.6
25.0
26.2
25.2
24.2

Mean 25.32 ± 0.81 mg (SEM $= 0.27$ mg).

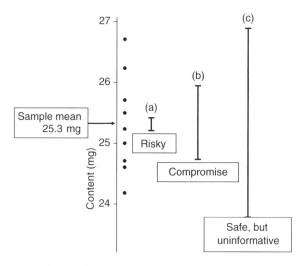

Figure 5.1 How wide a confidence interval for mean imipramine content in tablets?

5.2.1 A compromise is needed

In reality we need to use an interval that is wide enough to provide reasonable confidence that it will include the true population mean, without being so wide as to cease to be informative [e.g. interval (b) in Figure 5.1]. The generally accepted compromise is the so called '95 per cent confidence interval'.

5.3 What do we mean by '95 per cent' confidence?

The concept of being 95 per cent confident that an interval includes the population mean is difficult to comprehend in terms of a single case. After all, an interval is either 100 per cent right (it does include the population mean) or it is 100 per cent wrong. It cannot be 95 per cent correct! However, the concept makes perfectly good sense if viewed in terms of a long series. Imagine a scientist who regularly makes sets of measurements and then expresses the results as 95 per cent confidence intervals for the mean. The width of the intervals is calculated so that 19 out every 20 will include the true population mean. In the remaining twentieth case, an unusually unrepresentative sample generates an interval that fails to include it.

5.3.1 Other levels of confidence

It is possible to calculate other confidence intervals, e.g. 90 per cent or 98 per cent confidence intervals. If we routinely used 90 per cent CIs, we would have to accept being wrong on 10 per cent of occasions, whereas with 98 per cent CIs, we would be wrong only 2 per cent of the time. However, there is a downside to using higher levels of confidence, such as 98 per cent – the intervals have to be wider to provide that extra bit of assurance. In the real world, intervals for anything other than 95 per cent confidence are not commonly met.

5.4 Calculating the interval width

We have already identified the factors that govern the reliability of a sample – variability within the data and the sample size (Chapter 4). It is these same factors that influence the width of a 95 per cent confidence interval

5.4.1 Variability in the data

We know that a high SD tends to spoil samples. So, if the SD is large, our sample will be relatively unreliable and the true population mean might be considerably higher or lower than our sample suggests. We will therefore have to set the interval relatively wide to ensure that we include the real population mean.

5.4.2 Sample size

With larger samples we will get estimates that are closer and closer to the truth, so we can afford to make the interval narrower. Figure 5.2 summarizes the situation. The plus sign indicates that an increase in SD will lead to a wider interval and the minus sign that increasing the sample size will reduce its width.

● **Width of confidence intervals**

Greater SDs give wider intervals.
Greater sample sizes give narrower intervals.

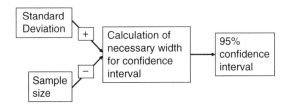

Figure 5.2   Calculation of the width of the 95 per cent confidence interval for the mean

Table 5.2 Generic output from calculation of 95 per cent CI for mean imipramine content in tablets

95% CI for mean: imipramine

n	Mean	SD	SEM	95% CI lower limit	95% CI upper limit
9	25.32	0.807	0.269	24.70	25.94

5.4.3 Using statistical packages to obtain 95 per cent confidence intervals

With most packages you will simply enter the data into a column, call up the appropriate routine and identify the column containing the data. You will then be supplied with a point estimate for the mean and the upper and lower limits of the confidence interval. Good old Excel and its Data Analysis tool half does the job: it provides a figure that needs to be added to/subtracted from the mean to obtain the limits of the interval.

For the imipramine tablets, Table 5.2 shows confidence limits of 24.70 and 25.94 mg. Therefore, we can state, with 95 per cent confidence, that if we returned to this batch of tablets and took larger and larger samples, the mean imipramine content would eventually settle down to some figure no less than 24.70 mg and no greater than 25.94 mg. This can be conveniently presented visually as in Figure 5.3. The dot indicates the point estimate and the horizontal bar represents the extent of the 95 per cent confidence interval.

5.5 A long series of samples and 95 per cent confidence intervals

Figure 5.4 shows simulated samples of nine tablets taken from a large batch, for which the true mean imipramine content is 25.0 ± 1.0 mg ($\pm$ SD). Each horizontal bar represents the 95 per cent confidence interval from one of the samples. Out of the 30 samples, we would expect 95 per cent to produce intervals that include the true population mean and the remainder (one or two cases) will be unusually misleading

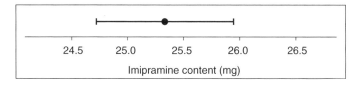

Figure 5.3 The 95 per cent confidence interval for the mean imipramine content among the population of tablets, based upon our sample

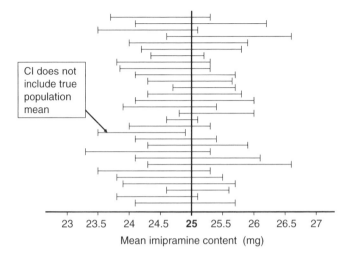

Figure 5.4 Simulation of repeated 95 per cent CIs for mean imipramine content of 30 samples. The population mean is known to be 25.0 mg

samples that lead to false intervals. That is pretty much what we see. There is just the one sample with a very low mean, that produced a misleading outcome. Notice that, even with the one interval that is technically incorrect, the true population mean is only marginally outside the interval. These confidence intervals are almost never seriously misleading.

🗝️ 95 per cent CI is a good compromise

The 95 per cent CIs have stood the test of time, providing a good compromise. They are narrow enough to be informative, but are almost never seriously misleading.

5.6 How sensitive is the width of the confidence interval to changes in the SD, the sample size or the required level of confidence?

5.6.1 Changing the SD

Figure 5.5 shows what happens to the width of the confidence interval if we change the SD of the data, but keep the sample size constant at 9. We had already anticipated that, as the SD increases, the interval will have to be widened. The relationship is simply linear in nature. Doubling the SD doubles the width of the interval.

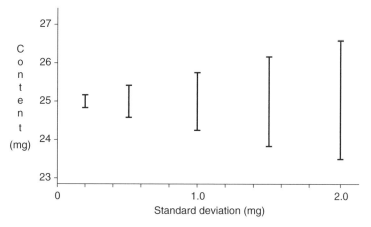

Figure 5.5   The 95 per cent confidence intervals for mean imipramine content. Population mean = 25 mg. Sample size = 9. The SD varies between ±0.2 and ±2 mg

5.6.2   Changing the sample size

Figure 5.6 looks at varying sample size while the SD is kept constant at ±1 mg. The relationship is dramatically sensitive at small sample sizes. With samples of less than about 10, any change in sample size greatly alters the width of the confidence interval. However, beyond 10, it is more of a struggle to reduce the width of the interval.

5.6.3   Changing the required level of confidence

Finally, Figure 5.7 shows the influence of the level of confidence required. The SD and sample size are kept constant, but the interval is calculated to provide anything

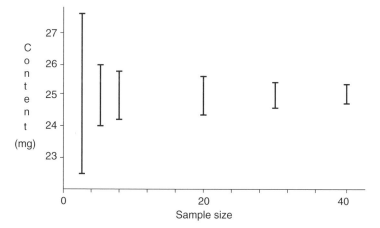

Figure 5.6   The 95 per cent confidence intervals for mean imipramine content. Population mean = 25 mg. The SD = ±1.0 mg. Sample size varies between 3 and 40

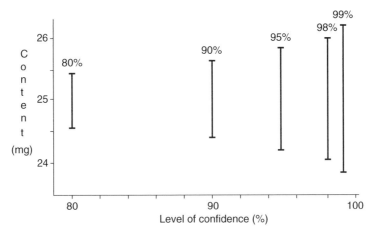

Figure 5.7 Confidence intervals for mean imipramine content. Population mean = 25 mg. SD = ±1.0 mg. Sample size = 9. The level of confidence varies between 80 and 99 per cent

between 80 and 99 per cent confidence. The width of the interval does increase if greater levels of confidence are required, but the relationship is not dramatic. The usual standard is 95 per cent confidence and any move up to 98 or down to 80 per cent confidence produces intervals that are not radically different.

The most striking conclusion from this section is that the biggest problems arise with very small samples. These lead to embarrassingly wide confidence intervals, and a relatively modest investment in a larger sample size would pay off handsomely.

⚊ The danger of small samples

Confidence intervals become wider with greater SDs, narrower with larger sample sizes and wider if higher levels of confidence are required. Most dramatically – small samples give horribly wide 95 per cent confidence intervals.

5.7 Two statements

The solution arrived at in this chapter is basically that we abandon any attempt to draw a single definitive conclusion, and instead we make two statements:

1. some conclusion about the population;

2. an assessment of the reliability of the first statement.

Our conclusion was that the population mean lies within a stated range and then we can say that 95 per cent of such statements are correct. This sets a pattern that we will see throughout statistics. All of the procedures that we will be looking at include this crucial stage of providing an objective assessment of the reliability of any conclusion that might be drawn.

 Assessing the reliability of our conclusions

Statistics never draws any absolute conclusions. It will offer an opinion and then back that up with a measure of that conclusion's reliability. It is a very grown up science, putting behind it the dubious certainties of childhood.

5.8 One-sided 95 per cent confidence intervals

The procedure we have followed so far actually entails making two claims as we have established both maximum and minimum limits for the mean. It has been emphasized that there is a 5 per cent chance of error. That overall 5 per cent hazard is split between two smaller risks – the maximum might be wrong or the minimum might be wrong. We refer to such a procedure as 'two-sided' or 'two-tailed'.

 Two-sided 95 per cent confidence intervals – two claims

1. The true population mean is no *less* than some stated figure (2.5 per cent chance that this is false).

2. The true population mean is no *greater* than some stated figure (2.5 per cent chance that this is false).

However, there are circumstances where only one of the above claims is actually of practical relevance. For example if we have manufactured a batch of crude drug for sale, the purchaser will demand some statement as to its minimum purity, but will hardly insist that we guarantee that it does not contain more than a particular amount of the authentic material. What we can do in such a case is to calculate what is initially a 90 per cent confidence interval for true drug content, which will generate two statements:

- Drug content is no less than this figure (5 per cent risk of error).

- Drug content is no greater than this other figure (5 per cent risk of error).

If we then only make the relevant claim and simply make no comment about possible values in the opposite direction, our total chance of error is only 5 per cent and we again have 95 per cent assurance that we are telling the truth. We then refer to this as a one-sided 95 per cent confidence interval.

If we apply this approach to the drug purity problem, in a long series of instances there will be three types of outcome. The true drug content may be:

1. below the minimum figure we quoted and we will have misled the customer and caused some annoyance (5 per cent of all cases);

2. within the two limits of the 90 per cent CI that was initially calculated; the customer is OK about that (90 per cent of all cases);

3. above the upper limit of our initial CI; we never made any claim as to maximum content and the customer certainly will not complain (5 per cent of all cases).

Whilst initially it might seem perverse to calculate a 90 per cent CI and then quote it as a 95 per cent CI, it is in fact perfectly fair so long as we quote only one of the confidence limits.

🔑 One-sided 95 per cent confidence intervals – one claim

Either
The true population mean is no *less* than some stated figure (5 per cent chance that this is false).
Or
The true population mean is no *greater* than some stated figure (5 per cent chance that this is false).

5.8.1 Using statistical packages to obtain one-sided confidence intervals

Most packages will produce one-sided intervals. There are two possible approaches:

- Find an option that allows you to select a one-sided interval in place of the default two-sided version. In this case you still request 95 per cent confidence.

- Stay with the two-sided version, but change the confidence level to 90 per cent. Then quote only the limit (max or min) that matches your requirements.

Using Excel, you would take the latter approach.

Table 5.3 Tetracyline content (per cent w/w) in 8 samples taken from a single batch

75.7
77.7
78.4
77.5
73.9
77.6
75.5
77.1

5.8.2 An example of a one-sided 95 per cent confidence interval – the purity of tetracycline

We have produced a batch of tetracycline and taken eight random samples of material from the batch. The results of analyses of the material are shown in Table 5.3. The potential purchaser requires a statement as to the minimum content of authentic material.

Using either of the approaches shown above should yield a lower limit for a one-sided 95 per cent confidence interval of 75.7 per cent tetracycline. This is the figure we can quote to a potential purchaser, knowing that there is only a 5 per cent risk that the true content might be any lower.

5.8.3 Visual presentation of one sided confidence intervals

Figure 5.8 shows a useful way to present one-sided confidence intervals. The idea is to emphasize the fact that we have established a definite lower limit, but are making no comment concerning how great the value might be. The figure also shows a normal two-sided 95 per cent CI for the same data; it places limits both above and below the mean.

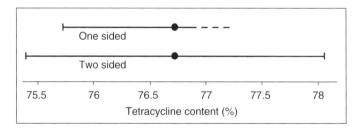

Figure 5.8 One and two-sided 95 per cent confidence intervals for the mean tetracycline content for a batch of product

5.8.4   A one-sided confidence limit is closer to the mean

Figure 5.8 also shows that, when a one-sided interval is calculated, the one limit that is calculated is closer to the mean than the corresponding limit for a two-sided interval. This is related to the amount of risk we are taking. With the one-sided interval, we are prepared to take a 5 per cent risk that the true mean might be below the indicated figure, but with the two-sided interval, we can only allow a 2.5 per cent chance of error.

⚷ One-sided confidence intervals

One sided CIs are a natural way to provide assurance that a value is no greater than (or less than) some critical value.

5.9   The 95 per cent confidence interval for the difference between two treatments

Experimental work often concerns comparisons between two differently treated groups of people (or animals or objects). Frequently, we will determine the mean value for some measured end-point in each group and then look at the difference between these. However, our two mean values will almost certainly be based upon samples and each will be subject to the usual random sampling error. If we are estimating the difference between two imperfectly defined values, the calculated difference will also be subject to sampling error. There is an obvious role for the 95 per cent CI for the difference between two means. Figure 5.9 shows a typical case, where we are comparing plasma cholesterol levels in two groups.

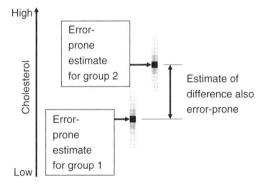

Figure 5.9   Uncertainty when estimating the difference between two sample means

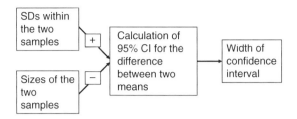

Figure 5.10   Calculation of the width of the 95 per cent confidence interval for the difference between two means

The error in estimating the difference will depend upon the imprecision of the two samples. If we have reliable estimates for mean cholesterol in both groups, then our estimate of the difference will also be reliable, but if both initial figures are imprecise, the calculated difference will be similarly woolly. We already know that the precision of the two samples depends upon their size and the variability of the data within each sample. Therefore, Figure 5.10 shows that the calculation of a 95 per cent confidence interval for the difference between two means will depend upon the SDs within the two samples (greater SDs bring more uncertainty and wider intervals) and the sizes of our samples (larger samples give greater precision and narrower intervals).

Any decent statistical package (not XL) will perform the calculation of such a confidence interval, but it will generally be presented as a so-called 't-test'. We will not consider the use of computers to produce this calculation any further at this juncture, but it lies at the heart of the next chapter.

> ## 🔑 Confidence interval for the difference between two means
>
> A 95 per cent confidence interval for the difference between two means can be calculated by taking account of the size of the two samples and their SDs.

5.10 The need for data to follow a normal distribution and data transformation

Many of the statistical methods we will look at are based on an assumption that the data follow a normal distribution. The standard method of calculating a 95 per cent CI is among these. It is generally accepted that, if the distribution of data is approximately (but not perfectly) normal, the resulting 95 per cent CI will not be unduly misleading. The term 'robust' is used to express this ability to perform acceptably even with moderately imperfect data. However, when data are grossly non-normal, even robust methods can lead to silly conclusions. In this section we will look at a problem case and see how we can circumvent the difficulty.

5.10.1 Pesticide residues in foxglove leaves

Crops of foxglove leaves have been collected for the extraction of the heart drug digoxin. The crops were from widely scattered sites. All have been analysed for contamination by a pesticide. The results are shown in the first column of Table 5.4

Figure 5.11(a) shows a histogram of this data and they are obviously not remotely normally distributed. There is a very strong positive skew arising because a few sites have values far above the main cluster and these cannot be balanced by similarly low values, as they would be negative concentrations.

We could simply turn a blind eye to this non-normality and proceed to generate a 95 per cent CI in the usual way and the results would be a mean of 95.9 with confidence limits of −23.1 to +215.0 ng/g. These are shown in Figure 5.12(a). The result is clearly nonsensical – the true population mean could not possibly take the sort of negative value implied by the lower limit of the confidence interval.

Table 5.4 Pesticide residues in 20 crops of foxglove leaves (ng/g leaf)

Concentration	Log of concentration
31.9	1.503
89.8	1.953
31.8	1.502
105.6	2.024
8.5	0.929
2.1	0.322
1.5	0.176
94.4	1.975
2.1	0.322
2.7	0.431
21.4	1.330
12.1	1.083
5.7	0.756
267.6	2.428
88.4	1.946
7.4	0.869
1.7	0.230
1141.8	3.058
0.5	−0.301
1.9	0.279

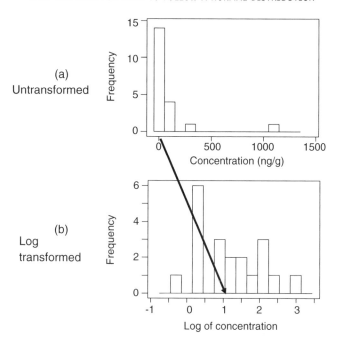

Figure 5.11 Log transformation of pesticide concentrations

🔑 Non-normal data

Data deviating dramatically from a normal distribution can produce severely misleading or even nonsensical confidence intervals.

5.10.2 The log transform

A well-established solution to such problems is to transform the data by taking logarithms of the original values. The log transformed data are shown in the second

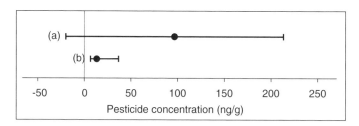

Figure 5.12 The 95 per cent confidence interval for mean pesticide content calculated (a) directly or (b) via log transformation

column of Table 5.4. (The logs used in this case are simple base 10 logs.) Figure 5.11(b) shows that with log transformation we have a far more symmetrically distributed data set. The reason for this is that the main cluster of values is around 10 ng/g. With the untransformed data, this main cluster lies at the extreme left-hand side of a scale going from 0 to 1500 ng/g. However, when we transform the data, values of 10 are transformed to log (10), which equals 1. Such values are then close to the middle of a scale going from −1 to 3. The arrow on Figure 5.12 shows the main cluster of values moving to the centre of the distribution thereby improving its symmetry.

We then calculate a mean and confidence interval using these log transformed values. The mean is 1.141, but as this was calculated from the logs of the data, we need to take the antilog to get the real mean. The mean is then antilog (1.141) = 13.8 ng/g. Similarly, the limits for the confidence interval (0.723 and 1.558) need to be transformed back to their antilogs (5.28 and 36.14 ng/g). These are then shown in Figure 5.12(b). The results now make sense with both limits being positive figures.

> ## ⊶⊙ Log transform
>
> The log transform will often convert badly positively skewed data to a reasonably normal distribution.

5.10.3   Arithmetic and geometric means

The mean value obtained varied according to the method of calculation. By the direct method it was 95.9, but using the log transformation it was only 13.8 ng/g. We distinguish between these two values as being the 'arithmetic' and 'geometric' means.

> ## ⊶⊙ Arithmetic and geometric means
>
> The arithmetic mean is calculated directly from the data.
> The geometric mean is calculated via log transformation of the data.

With normally distributed data the arithmetic and geometric means would be equal, but with positively skewed data the arithmetic mean is always greater than the geometric mean.

5.10.4   Log transform gives asymmetrical limits

The 95 per cent CI [Figure 5.12(b)] obtained via the log transform is markedly asymmetrical and this is characteristic of CIs obtained in this way.

5.10.5 Other transformations

A whole range of other transformations have been recommended for particular purposes. Two that are met with on occasions are the square-root and square transforms.

Square-root transform The log transform has a dramatic effect upon the data and is sometimes too powerful: positively skewed data may be transformed into equally troublesome, negatively skewed data! The square-root transform has the same basic effect as the log transform – pushing the mode to the right. However, it is often less extreme and may be preferable in cases of moderate positive skew. As the name implies, we just take the square-roots of the problem data.

The square transform Negative skew tends to be a lot rarer than the positive form, but when it does raise its ugly head, transforming the data by squaring all the values may help.

5.11 Chapter summary

A confidence interval for the mean is derived from sample data and allows us to establish a range within which we may assert that the population mean is likely to lie. In the case of 95 per cent CIs, such statements will be correct on 95 per cent of occasions. In the remaining 5 per cent of cases, particularly misleading samples will produce intervals that are either too high or too low and do not include the true population mean.

The width of the confidence interval will depend upon the SD for the sample, the size of the sample and the degree of confidence required. The width is especially dependent upon sample size – small samples lead to very wide intervals. One-sided confidence intervals can be used to specify a value that the population mean is unlikely to exceed (or be less than).

A 95 per cent CI for the difference between two sample means can be calculated by taking account of the size of the two samples and the standard deviations within each sample. Data to be used to calculate a CI for the mean should be at least approximately normally distributed. Severely non-normal data can lead to misleading intervals.

Data that are markedly positively skewed can sometimes be restored to normality by log transformation, thereby allowing the calculation of a geometric mean and 95 per cent CI.

6

The two-sample *t*-test (1). Introducing hypothesis tests

This chapter will ...

- Introduce hypothesis tests

- Describe the use of the two-sample *t*-test to determine whether there is a real difference in a measured (interval scale) end-point between two sets of observations

- Describe null and alternative hypotheses

- Describe the use of the two-sample *t*-test to generate a 95 per cent CI for the difference between the two means

- Show how the confidence interval is used to diagnose whether there is sufficient evidence of a difference

- Set out the characteristics that data should fulfil if it is to be subjected to a two-sample *t*-test

- Introduce the statistical use of the term 'significance'

- Explore the aspects of the data that will determine whether a significant result is obtained

Essential Statistics for the Pharmaceutical Sciences   Philip Rowe
© 2007 John Wiley & Sons, Ltd   ISBN 9780470 03470 5 (HB)   ISBN 9780 470 03468 2 (PB)

- Introduce the synonymous terms 'false positive' and 'type I error'

- Show the use of 'alpha' to report the risk of a false positive

6.1 The two sample *t*-test – an example of a hypothesis test

6.1.1 What do these tests do?

At first sight, data may seem to suggest that a drug treatment changes people's cholesterol levels or that high salt consumption is associated with high blood pressure, etc. However, we always need to use a statistical test to determine how convincing the evidence actually is. Such tests are known generically as 'hypothesis tests'.

The first experimental design we are going to consider involves the measurement of the same end-point in two groups of people, rats, tablets (or whatever). We calculate the mean value of the end-point in each group and then want to test whether there is convincing evidence of a difference between the two mean values. The procedure we use is a two-sample *t*-test, the term 'two-sample' reflecting the fact that we are comparing two distinct samples of individuals.

The test is also known as the 'independent samples *t*-test' or the 'Student *t*-test'. The use of numerous apparently distinct names for exactly the same test is a handy device used by statisticians to keep everybody else in a constant state of uncertainty.

6.1.2 An example – does rifampicin change the rate of elimination of theophylline?

It is known that the antibiotic rifampicin increases the amount of drug metabolizing enzyme present in the liver and consequently increases the rate of elimination of a wide range of other drugs. This experiment is designed to detect whether rifampicin affects the metabolic removal of the anti-asthma drug theophylline. Any such interaction could be of real practical importance. A marked increase in the elimination of theophylline would result in inadequate treatment of the patient's asthma.

In the experiment, there are two groups of 15 subjects. For the first group, each individual was pre-treated with oral rifampicin (600 mg daily for 10 days). The other group acted as a control, receiving only placebo pre-treatment. All subjects then received an intravenous injection of theophylline (3 mg/kg). A series of blood samples was obtained after the theophylline injections, and analysed for drug content. The efficiency of removal of theophylline was reported as a clearance value. Any increase in clearance would be interpreted as evidence that

Table 6.1 Clearance of theophylline (ml/min/kg) for
control subjects and for those pre-treated with rifampicin

	Control	Treated
	0.81	1.15
	1.06	1.28
	0.43	1.00
	0.54	0.95
	0.68	1.06
	0.56	1.15
	0.45	0.72
	0.88	0.79
	0.73	0.67
	0.43	1.21
	0.46	0.92
	0.43	0.67
	0.37	0.76
	0.73	0.82
	0.93	0.82
Mean	0.633	0.931 ml/min/kg
SD	0.216	0.202 ml/min/kg

rifampicin had increased the ability of the liver to eliminate this drug. The results
are shown in Table 6.1 and Figure 6.1. (The units of clearance are millilitres of
blood cleared of drug every minute per kilogram of body weight.) In our samples,
the mean clearance is about 50 per cent greater in the treated group compared
with the controls.

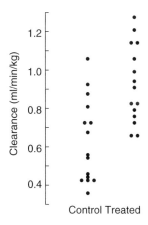

Figure 6.1 Theophylline clearance (ml/min/kg) in controls and in subjects pre-treated with
rifampicin

6.1.3   Null and alternative hypotheses

If rifampicin had no effect on the liver, the mean clearance in two very large groups of control and treated subjects would be virtually identical. However, with limited samples like these, both samples would probably yield imperfect estimates and their two means would almost certainly differ even in the absence of any real drug effect.

⚖ An apparent difference even in the absence of any real treatment effect

Samples are always subject to random error and control and treated samples are unlikely to produce identical means, even when a treatment has absolutely no real effect.

There are therefore two possible explanations for the difference in clearance between our two samples; it could have arisen by sheer chance or it could be indicative of a real and consistent effect. The two possible explanations are formally called 'null' and 'alternative' hypotheses. Remember that at this stage these are simply two competing theories. As yet, we have not decided which should be accepted.

- *Null hypothesis* – there is no real effect. The apparent difference arose from random sampling error. If we could investigate larger and larger numbers of subjects, the mean clearances for the two groups would eventually settle down to the same value. In stat speak 'the difference between the population mean clearances is zero'.

- *Alternative hypothesis* – there is a real effect and this is what caused the difference between the mean clearances. If we investigated larger and larger numbers of subjects, the results would continue to confirm a change in clearance. Also translatable into stat speak as 'the difference between the population mean clearances is *not* zero'.

All hypothesis tests start by setting out appropriate null and alternative hypotheses such as those above.

⚖ Null hypothesis

The statistical wet blanket. Whatever interesting feature has been noted in our sample (a change in an end-point or a relationship between two sets of data) is assumed not to be present in the general population. The apparent change or relationship is claimed to be due solely to random sampling error.

> ⚷ Alternative hypothesis
>
> The logical alternative to whatever the null hypothesis claims. It will claim that the effect or relationship seen in the sample is perfectly real, i.e. present in the wider population.

To follow the analysis, it is particularly important to understand the mechanism implied by the null hypothesis. Figure 6.2 will be used to describe these alleged events. A vertical scale shows theophylline clearances. Each circle (open or solid) represents a member of the population. The data form normal distributions (but these are shown turned at right angles to the usual orientation).

According to the null hypothesis, the two populations have identical means (as shown). We have then selected some individuals for inclusion in our random sample (solid circles). The null hypothesis assumes that our samples were both somewhat unrepresentative, leading to an apparently lower mean among the controls than among the treated subjects. At the end of the experiment, all we would actually see would be the two samples with their differing means.

The alternative hypothesis (Figure 6.3) is much simpler. There really is a difference – the mean clearance among pre-treated individuals is greater than that among the controls – and the difference between our samples merely reflects that fact.

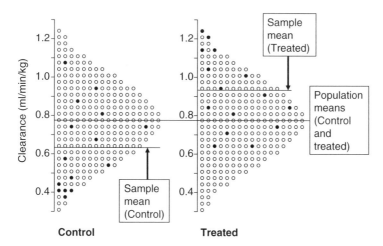

Figure 6.2 Null hypothesis: random sampling error produced the appearance of an effect, although none was really present

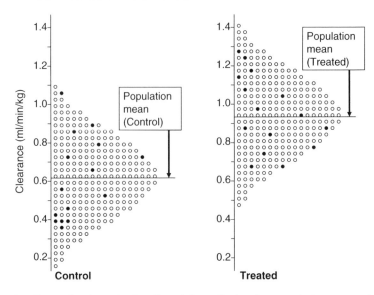

Figure 6.3 Alternative hypothesis: rifampicin really has increased clearance values – no need to assume sampling error

6.1.4 Using the test to generate the 95 per cent confidence interval for the difference between the two treatments

The function of the *t*-test is to assess the credibility of the null hypothesis. Its principal function is to generate a 95 per cent CI for the difference between the two treatments. (We have already met the idea of a 95 per cent CI for the difference between means in Section 5.9.)

From this point on, you can pretty well kiss Excel goodbye. For reasons that will be clarified in Chapter 9, its implementation of the two-sample *t*-test is highly undesirable.

In most packages, you will enter the data from both samples into a single column of a data sheet and then set up a second column that contains labels indicating which sample each value belongs to. With the theophylline clearance data, you would place

Table 6.2 Generic output from a two-sample *t*-test comparing theophylline clearances in rifampicin treated and control subjects

Two sample *t*-test	
Mean (Rif_treated)	0.931
Mean (control)	0.633
Difference (Rif_treated − control)	+0.298
95 per cent CI difference	+0.142 to +0.455
P	0.001

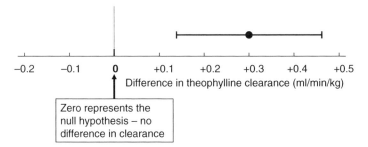

Figure 6.4 The 95 per cent confidence interval for the difference in theophylline clearance between control and rifampicin treated subjects

the 30 clearance values in one column and then, in another column, the first 15 cells would contain a code indicating a result from a rifampicin-treated subject result and the next 15 would contain a code indicating a control. In some packages you will have to use numbers to code the two groups in which case '0' is commonly used for controls and '1' for treated individuals, but any two numbers could be used. Many packages allow meaningful text labels such as 'Rif_treated' and 'Control'. To perform the test you will simply identify which column contains the data and which the treatment codes. In some packages, there is an option to enter the data for each sample in separate columns and then identify the two columns of data.

6.1.5   Is the null hypothesis credible?

Parts of the output (See Table 6.2) may not be immediately familiar, but will be explained later. The key part at the moment is the 95 per cent CI for the difference (expressed as clearance for treated subjects minus that for the controls) with limits of +0.142 and +0.455 ml/min/kg. It is useful to represent this pictorially, as in Figure 6.4

Figure 6.4 tells us that, if we were to collect more and more data, the difference in clearance would not necessarily remain at the point estimate of +0.298 ml/min/kg that our small samples yielded. Ultimately we might find the true difference is actually as small as +0.142 or as large as +0.455 ml/min/kg.

The key point is that it is pretty obvious that the null hypothesis (with its claim of a difference of zero) is difficult to believe – zero lies well outside the 95 per cent CI. Since the null hypothesis now looks so shaky, the balance shifts in favour of accepting the alternative hypothesis that rifampicin really does cause a change in theophylline clearance.

6.1.6   The generalities of the two-sample *t*-test

The two-sample *t*-test is a general procedure applicable to any situation where we have two samples, the same measured end-point has been determined for both and the question being posed is whether there is convincing evidence of a change in the

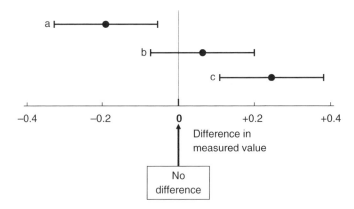

Figure 6.5 General interpretation of the results of a two-sample *t*-test

end-point. The general interpretation of the results that we might obtain from a two-sample *t*-test are shown in Figure 6.5.

Two of the confidence intervals (a and c) would be interpreted as providing evidence of a difference. In the upper case (a) we see a convincing decrease and in (c) a convincing increase. In the middle case (b), we would have to conclude that the evidence is not adequate to permit any positive conclusions – there is a real possibility that the treatment has no effect on whatever we were measuring, since a zero difference is included within the confidence interval.

⚷ Is there evidence of an effect?

If the CI *includes* zero, the null hypothesis that the treatment produces no effect is credible. Nothing has been proved.

If the CI *excludes* zero, we have worthwhile evidence that there is an experimental effect.

6.2 'Significance'

Where the confidence interval for a difference excludes zero, the data obviously provide considerable support for the existence of a real difference and the results are granted the status of being 'significant'. The original choice of this word was very canny. It tells us that the evidence is worthy of note and should be added to whatever other evidence is available. Unfortunately, many slip into the lazy habit of simply assuming that, if the current set of results are significant, then the case is proven – period. The correct interpretation of statistical significance is discussed more fully in Chapter 11.

When zero is within the 95 per cent CI, the results are described as 'non-significant'. The use of 'insignificant' as the opposite of significant looks uneducated.

⚏ Significant and non-significant

If the evidence is 'significant', it is strong enough to merit being added to whatever body of knowledge already exists. It does not mean that we should blindly accept the current result.

'Non-significant' implies that the evidence is weak and will have little influence upon our thinking.

6.3 The risk of a false positive finding

6.3.1 What would happen if there was no real effect?

A major requirement of any statistical test is that it should provide protection against concluding that there is a real effect in circumstances where none really exists. This protection is considered below.

If the truth were that rifampicin actually had no effect at all (true mean effect = zero) and we repeatedly carried out the previous experiment, then we would anticipate the sort of results seen in Figure 6.6. Out of 20 experiments, 19 would be successful – the 95 per cent CI would include the true mean change (none) and we

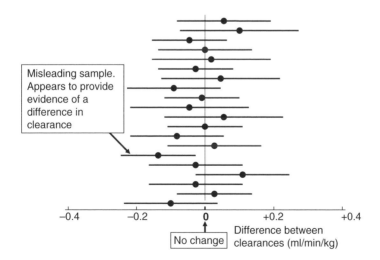

Figure 6.6 Repeated determinations of the 95 per cent CI for the difference in theophylline clearance between control and rifampicin-treated subjects, assuming that there is actually no effect

would correctly conclude that there is no convincing evidence of an effect. In the one remaining experiment, we get an unfortunate coincidence of high values in one sample and low values in the other, leading to apparently convincing evidence of a difference, (In this case, there seems to be a reduction in clearance). In that one case, we would make a false diagnosis. Typically, when there is no real effect present, we will be fooled on just one out of 20 (5 per cent) of occasions.

Cases where there is no real effect but we erroneously conclude that there is are called 'false positives'. Another name for these is a 'type I error'.

⚷ 'False positives' or 'type I errors'

If there is no real effect of the treatment we are investigating, but we happen to obtain particularly misleading samples, we may wrongly conclude that there is adequate evidence of an effect. In that case, we have generated a 'false positive' or 'type I error'.

6.3.2 Alpha

The Greek letter alpha 'α' is used to represent this small residual risk of a false positive. Alpha obviously depends upon what confidence interval is inspected. In the case of the standard 95 per cent CI, the remaining risk is $100 - 95 = 5$ per cent. However, if we were particularly anxious to avoid the risk of a false positive, we might calculate a 98 per cent CI and only declare a positive finding if that wider interval excluded zero. In that case alpha would be only 2 per cent.

⚷ α – the rate of false positives

Whenever we investigate a situation where there is no real difference present, α is the risk that we will generate a false positive finding. With the usual 95 per cent CIs, α is 5 per cent.

6.4 What factors will influence whether or not we obtain a significant outcome?

Figure 6.5 made the point that we are looking to see if the 95 per cent confidence interval crosses (and therefore includes) the zero line. Two things influence the likelihood of a significant outcome and these are shown in Figures 6.7 and 6.8.

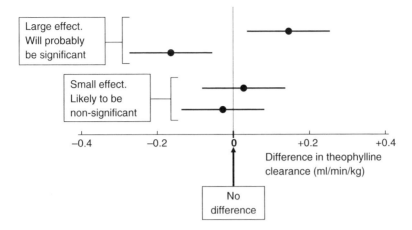

Figure 6.7 The size of the experimental effect and the likelihood of obtaining a significant outcome

Figure 6.7 shows the influence of the size of the experimental effect. If the mean clearances differ to only a very small extent (as in the two lower cases in Figure 6.7), then the 95 per cent confidence interval will probably overlap zero, bringing a non-significant result. However, with a large effect (as in the two upper cases), the confidence interval is displaced well away from zero and will not overlap it.

Figure 6.8 shows the effect of the width of the confidence interval. We know that the interval width depends upon the variability (SD) of the data being considered and the number of observations available. Therefore, if the theophylline clearances are fairly consistent and large numbers of subjects have been studied,

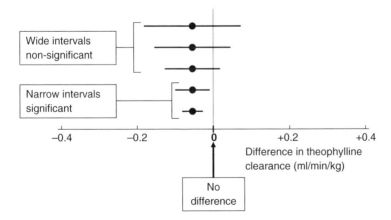

Figure 6.8 Width of the confidence interval and likelihood of obtaining a significant outcome

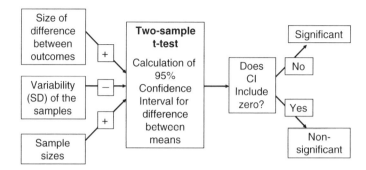

Figure 6.9   Factors influencing the outcome of a two-sample *t*-test

the interval will be narrow (as at the bottom of the figure) and the result significant. At the other extreme, if the clearances are highly variable and numbers of subjects small, the interval will be wide, as at the top of the figure and the result non-significant.

In summary, whether or not a significant outcome arises depends upon:

- the size of the experimental effect;

- the width of the confidence interval, which in turn depends upon the variability in the data and the sample size.

This is summarized in Figure 6.9. In this figure, the plus and minus signs are used to indicate the effect each factor has on the chances of a significant outcome.

- A large experimental effect will increase the chances of a significant result. Hence the plus sign.

- A large SD will widen the confidence interval and increase the danger of overlap and so significance becomes less likely, so this gets a minus sign.

- A large sample size will make the confidence interval narrower and so reduce the danger of overlap – making significance more likely – so this gets a plus sign.

⚷ Aspects taken into account by the two-sample *t*-test

The two-sample *t*-test takes account of the apparent size of the experimental effect, the SDs of the samples and the sample sizes. It then combines all of these to determine whether the data are statistically significant.

An important aspect of the two-sample *t*-test is the ability to off-set the three relevant aspects against one another. A couple of examples are set out below:

- If an experimental effect is present but is small in size, this makes it harder (but not impossible) to detect. What we would need to do is to strengthen the other two factors as much as possible. The amount of control we have over the variability in the data is pretty limited, so the main recourse would be to larger sample sizes. It does not matter how small the effect is; it is always possible to detect it if we can obtain sufficiently large samples.

- In the more comfortable scenario of a large experimental effect and data with low SDs, we would have the luxury of being able to use samples and yet still obtain a significant result.

6.5 Requirements for applying a two-sample *t*-test

6.5.1 The two sets of data must approximate to normal distributions and have similar SDs

The data within each of the two samples should be drawn from populations that are normally distributed and have equal SDs. We have to be aware that the data we are dealing with are small samples. Judgements can be tricky. Even if populations adhere perfectly to the above requirements, small samples drawn from them are unlikely to have perfect, classic, bell-shaped distributions or to have exactly coincident SDs.

🔑 Assumption of normal distributions and equal SDs

The mathematical basis of the two-sample *t*-test assumes that the samples are drawn from populations that:

- are normally distributed;

- have equal SDs.

The test is quite robust, but where there is strong evidence of non-normality or unequal SDs, action is required. We may be able to convert the data to normality, for example by the use of a logarithmic transformation (introduced in Chapter 5). Alternatively, we may have to use an alternative type of test ('non-parametric') which does not require a normal distribution. These are discussed in Chapter 17.

Where the problem is solely one of unequal SDs, there is a minor variant of the test, 'Welch's approximate *t*', that does not have this requirement. In fact, in Minitab, this is the default test, and if you want the classical *t*-test, you will have to select it (see the web site for details).

⚷ The two-sample *t*-test is robust but there are limits

The two-sample *t*-test is robust, i.e. it will still function reasonably well with samples that are somewhat non-normally distributed. However, where data is severely non-normal, even this test will start to produce inappropriate conclusions. In that case, either transform the data to normality or use a non-parametric test.

6.6 Chapter summary

We have met our first 'hypothesis test'. The two-sample *t*-test is used to determine whether two samples have produced convincingly different mean values or whether the difference is small enough to be explained away as random sampling error. The data in each sample are assumed to be from populations that followed normal distributions and had equal SDs.

We create a null hypothesis that there is no real experimental effect and that for large samples, the mean value of the end-point is exactly the same for both treatments. According to this hypothesis, random sampling error is responsible for any apparent difference and with extended sampling the apparent difference would eventually evaporate.

The alternative hypothesis claims that there is a real effect and that there is a difference between the mean values for the two populations. If we took larger and larger samples the difference would continue to make itself apparent.

A 95 per cent CI for difference between the two means is used to determine whether the null hypothesis is reasonably credible. If the 95 per cent CI includes zero, the results are compatible with the null hypothesis and are declared 'non-significant'. If the 95 per cent CI excludes zero, we have worthwhile evidence against the null hypothesis and declare the results 'significant'.

The outcome of the test is governed by:

- size of the difference between the sample means (greater difference means significance more likely);

- SDs within the data (greater SDs means significance less likely);

- sample sizes (greater sample sizes means significance more likely).

If we investigate a situation where there is no real difference and test our data by constructing a 95 per cent CI, we know that there is 95 per cent assurance that our interval will include the true treatment effect of zero and that we will draw the appropriate conclusion that the data are non-significant. This leaves a residual 5 per cent risk that unusually misleading samples will apparently indicate significant evidence in favour of an effect. Such events are referred to as 'false positives' or 'type I errors'. The degree of risk of such an event is represented by the Greek letter alpha – α. If a 95 per cent CI is being used to test for significance, $\alpha = 5$ per cent.

7

The two-sample *t*-test (2). The dreaded *P* value

This chapter will . . .

- Explain the information conveyed by *P* values

- Describe how *P* values can be used to determine statistical significance

- Describe how *P* values should be reported

- Review how useful (or otherwise) *P* values actually are

7.1 Measuring how significant a result is

In the last chapter, we saw how experimental results could be tested for statistical significance. The outcome was simply dichotomous – the results were either 'significant' or 'non-significant'. However, one could imagine a hypothetical series of outcomes such as those seen in Figure 7.1.

Outcomes (a)–(d) and (f)–(i) would all be judged significant and yet there are clearly considerable differences among them. Outcomes such as (d) or (f) are just barely significant, with zero only slightly outside the confidence interval, whereas for

Essential Statistics for the Pharmaceutical Sciences   Philip Rowe
© 2007 John Wiley & Sons, Ltd   ISBN 9780 470 03470 5 (HB)   ISBN 9780 470 03468 2 (PB)

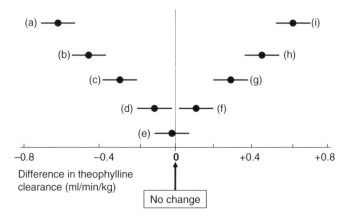

Figure 7.1   Various hypothetical outcomes for the effect of rifampicin on the clearance of theophylline

(a) or (i), the interval is well away from zero and the data are very clearly significant. The ancient statisticians who founded the methods of hypothesis testing hit upon a way to quantitate the level of significance. The underlying logic takes some thinking about, so concentrate hard . . .

7.2   *P* values

We need to consider hypothetically what would happen if we investigated a treatment that had absolutely no effect. In particular, we calculate the risk that we might obtain a result as impressive as the one we actually observed. That likelihood is then quoted as the *P* value.

The *P* value can then be used as a measure of the strength of the evidence – the lower the *P* value, the more unlikely it is that such results would arise by sheer chance and so the stronger the evidence. An outcome such as (e) would be very likely to arise with a treatment that has no real effect, so it has a high *P* value and provides virtually no useful evidence. Result (d) in Figure 8.1, would arise relatively rarely as the interval fails to include zero; however such 'near misses' are not that rare and its *P* value would be a few percent (but less than 5 per cent) – moderately strong evidence of an effect. The likelihood of obtaining an outcome such as (a) or (i) with a treatment that does not really produce any real change would be extremely low, so its *P* value would be some minute fraction of a per cent. Such a result would provide very strong evidence in favour of an effect.

A strict understanding of *P* needs to take account of two things:

- When considering an effect of a given size, we need to describe the likelihood of events that are not only exactly equal in size to the one we observed but also those more extreme. So, for outcome (d), we want to describe the likelihood of obtaining that exact result *or something even more extreme* such as (a), (b) or (c).

- When determining the risk of an event such as (d), we must remember that outcome (f) would also arise with equal likelihood and would provide equally impressive evidence of an effect (albeit in the opposite direction). When determining *P* we must therefore calculate the likelihood of an appropriately large difference *in either direction*.

Our final definition of the *P* value is therefore:

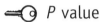 *P* value

P is the likelihood that, even with a treatment that has no real effect, we would observe an effect (positive or negative) as extreme as (or more extreme than) the one actually observed.

7.3 Two ways to define significance?

For no particular reason, the founding fathers of statistics decided to declare results 'significant' if the associated *P* value was less than 5 per cent (0.05). At this point you might feel we have a problem – we now seem to have two criteria of significance:

- If the 95 per cent confidence interval for the size of the experimental effect excludes zero, the result is significant.

- If the *P* value is less than 0.05, the result is significant.

However, although these two criteria sound very different, they are in fact mathematically equivalent. With any set of data, the outcome will either be significant by both criteria or non-significant by both. We will never be faced with the dilemma of one criterion indicating significance but not the other.

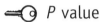 *P* values and significance

Results are rated as significant if *P* is less than 0.05. This criterion will always produce a verdict concordant with that based upon inspection of whether the 95 per cent CI for the effect size includes zero.

7.4 Obtaining the *P* value

Pretty well all statistical packages will include a *P* value as part of their out-put for the *t*-test. It was included as the last line in the generic output in Table 6.2, although its meaning was not explained at that stage.

Whatever package is used, the theophylline clearance data from the previous chapter should produce a *P* value of 0.001. This can be read as:

> If rifampicin actually had no effect on theophylline clearance, there would be only a 0.1 per cent (1 in 1000) chance that our samples would suggest an effect as great as (or greater than) the difference we actually observed.

As this data had already been declared significant on the basis of the 95 per cent CI for the size of the treatment effect, we would expect the *P* value to agree with this. The achieved *P* is indeed less than 0.05 and therefore significant.

⚬⊙ Reporting result in terms of the *P* value

The data provided significant evidence of a change in clearance ($P = 0.001$)

7.4.1 Very low *P* values

Where data are overwhelmingly significant, some statistical packages have a nasty habit of generating silly *P* values e.g. '$P = 0.000000012$'. Values as low as this are highly suspect, particularly as they would require our experimental data to adhere to a perfect normal distribution to an extent that we could never guarantee. The solution adopted in some statistical packages is a little brutal – they just round the result to a fixed number of decimal places and report in a format such as '$P = 0.000$'. This is also open to criticism as it could be read as a claim that there is a zero probability that such a result would arise by chance. This is never the case. If packages produce such output, it is probably best reported as '$P < 0.001$'

7.5 *P* values or 95 per cent confidence intervals?

Traditionally statistics books used to emphasize *P* values. This was probably because the manual calculation of whether or not *P* is less than 0.05 is quite manageable, but for many statistical tests, calculation of the exact limits of the 95 per cent CI can be pretty arduous. However, modern computer-based statistical packages remove that problem. Our choice of approach should now be based upon a consideration of what is best, not what involves the minimum of calculation steps. There are considerable arguments for preferring an inspection of the 95 per cent CI. These mainly arise because the P value only answers the question 'is there an effect?', whereas the 95 per cent CI answers that question, and additionally the question 'how great is the effect?' Chapter 9, in particular, will raise questions which can be answered only by inspecting the 95 per cent CI for the size of the experimental response. In these cases, the P value is at best useless and at worst downright misleading.

The P value may have passed its glory days but it is not yet dead and buried:

- It has some value in quantifying just how strong our evidence is. A P value < 0.001 tells us the evidence is very strong, whereas $P = 0.04$ indicates that the data are barely significant. Inspection of the CI provides a visual (but not quantitative) impression of the same information. An interval that stops just short of zero is significant (but only just) whereas an interval that is far removed from zero indicates much stronger evidence.

- For some of the statistical routines that we will look at later, there is no single CI that could encapsulate the overall significance of a data set, so computer packages only report the P value not a CI

This book will always emphasize the use of 95 per cent CIs wherever possible, but accept that in some circumstances, P is all we are going to get.

⊸○ *P* values – a dubious legacy?

In the past there has been an over-emphasis on P values. They are going to be around for a long time yet, but for many tests, P is less informative than the 95 per cent CI and it is the latter that should be focused upon.

7.6 Chapter summary

P values provide a way to express just how significant a finding is. The correct interpretation of P is:

> If the treatment we investigated actually produces no effect, the chances that we would obtain a result as impressive as (or more impressive than) the one we actually obtained, is P.

If the P value is less than 5 per cent (0.05), we interpret the result as statistically significant. The verdict will always be the same as that obtained by observing whether the 95 per cent CI for the difference between outcomes includes zero.

Very low *P* values should not be quoted as unjustifiably small figures. It is better to report these as being less than some appropriately small figure (e.g. $P < 0.001$).

The *P* value gives no information regarding the size of the experimental effect and is therefore, for many purposes, much less useful than the 95 per cent CI for the size of the difference. Where the latter is available, it should be emphasized rather than the *P* value.

8

The two-sample *t*-test (3). False negatives, power and necessary sample sizes

> ### *This chapter will* . . .
>
> - Describe 'false negatives' (type II errors), where we fail to detect a difference when one is actually present
>
> - Show how we use 'beta' to report the risk that we may fail to detect a difference and 'power' to report the level of assurance that we will detect it
>
> - Consider the aspects of an experiment that determine its power
>
> - Expound the need to plan rationally how large our samples should be
>
> - Show how to calculate the necessary sample sizes for an experiment that will be analysed by a two-sample *t*-test
>
> - Suggest that experiments should be planned to be large enough (and therefore sufficiently sensitive) to detect any difference that would be of practical significance, but that resources should not be squandered trying to detect trivially small differences

Essential Statistics for the Pharmaceutical Sciences   Philip Rowe
© 2007 John Wiley & Sons, Ltd   ISBN 9780 470 03470 5 (HB)   ISBN 9780 470 03468 2 (PB)

8.1 What else could possibly go wrong?

In the last two chapters we established that, in a situation where there is actually no experimental effect, we will correctly declare that the evidence is unconvincing 95 per cent of the time. This leaves us with a small (5 per cent) proportion of cases where the sample misleads us and we declare the evidence significant. We referred to these cases as 'false positives' or 'type I errors'. In this chapter we consider a new and quite different type of error.

8.1.1 False negatives – type II errors

One of the factors that feeds into the calculation of a two-sample *t*-test is the sample size. If we investigate a case where there is a real difference, but use too small a sample size, this may widen the 95 per cent confidence interval to the point where it overlaps zero. In that case, the results would be declared non-significant. This is a different kind of error. We are now failing to detect an effect that actually is present. This is a 'false negative' or 'type II error'.

🔑 'False negative' = 'type II error'

Failure to detect a difference that genuinely is present.

8.1.2 The beta value

The beta value (β) does a similar job to the alpha value. It reports the rate of type II errors. However, matters are a little more complicated, because the chances of detecting an experimental effect very much depend on how large it is (see Figure 6.9). If a large effect is present, it will be easy to detect, but very small effects are much more elusive. Think about the clearance data in the last two chapters. If rifampicin had a minute effect upon theophylline clearance – say it reduced average clearance by 1 per cent – this would be almost impossible to detect and a type II error would be practically inevitable. In contrast, a very large change in clearance would be much easier to detect and a type II error would be less likely. Consequently, beta has to be defined in terms of the risk of failing to detect some stated size of experimental effect.

🔑 Beta

If a real difference *of a stated size* is present, then beta defines the risk that we might fail to detect it.

Table 8.1 Errors and truths

	Difference is not actually present	Difference is actually present
No difference detected	Correct	Type II error False negative (β)
Difference is detected	Type I error False positive (α)	Correct

The different types of error that can arise can be neatly summarized as in Table 8.1. Two of the possible outcomes are satisfactory. In the top left hand box, there is no effect and we declare the evidence to be non-significant, and in the bottom right hand box an effect is present and we declare the evidence to be significant. The two types of error are seen in the other two boxes. In the top right case, we fail to detect a difference and, in the lower left, we declare the evidence to be significant when there is no real difference.

8.2 Power

If beta is the chance that we will fail to detect a difference, then power is simply the opposite; it is the chances that we will successfully detect the difference.

 Power

If a difference *of a stated size* is present, then power defines the likelihood that we will detect it and declare the evidence statistically significant.

Power and beta are then simply related as:

$$Power = 100\% - \beta$$

So, if beta is 10 per cent, power would be 90 per cent.

8.2.1 The power curve

Power will be related to sample size. Figure 8.1 shows the underlying logic using the investigation of altered theophylline clearance as an example. At the top of the figure, small samples produce wide 95 per cent CIs which are almost certain to overlap zero, so there is little hope of significance. At the bottom of the figure, large samples

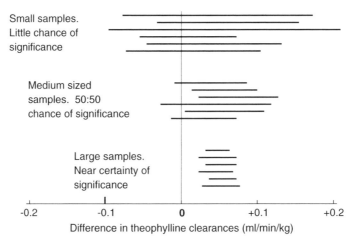

Small samples.
Little chance of
significance

Medium sized
samples. 50:50
chance of significance

Large samples.
Near certainty of
significance

-0.2   -0.1   0   +0.1   +0.2

Difference in theophylline clearances (ml/min/kg)

Figure 8.1   Effect of sample size upon the width of the 95 per cent CI for the difference in outcomes and hence on likelihood of statistical significance

produce narrow intervals and significance is practically guaranteed. However there is an intermediate situation where the outcome is unpredictable. With medium-sized samples, we may obtain a sample that happens to slightly understate the size of the difference in clearances and the CI crosses zero (non-significant), but the next sample suggests a greater difference and the result is significant.

Therefore, power increases with sample size. The relationship between sample size and power for our rifampicin/theophylline experiment is illustrated in Figure 8.2.

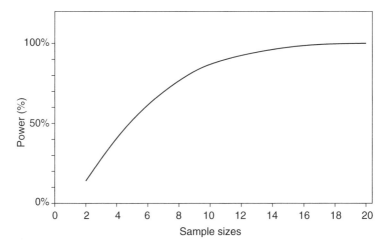

Figure 8.2   Power curve for the theophylline clearance experiment (assumes the true difference is an increase of 0.3 ml/min/kg and the SD among clearances is ±0.21 ml/min/kg)

This assumes that the true difference between the placebo and rifampicin-treated subjects is 0.3 ml/min/kg and that the SD of theophylline clearance is 0.21 ml/min/kg.

The figure shows that, with very small samples (less than 5), there would be little chance of detecting the change in clearance, but with larger samples (20 or more) we are almost certain to detect the effect. With sample size of 5 our chances of achieving a significant outcome are about 50:50. The sample size used in the our experiment introduced in Chapter 6 was 10, which provided a power of about 86 per cent.

8.2.2 Factors determining the power of an experiment

Power is influenced by four aspects of any experiment.

Size of difference that we are trying to detect   As described in Section 8.1.2, large differences are easier to detect than small ones and so the greater the difference we are trying to detect, the greater the power of our experiment.

Sample size   In the previous section we saw that sample size has a strong influence upon power. Greater sample sizes give greater power.

Variability of the data   We know that the width of the 95 per cent CI depends upon the variability of the data (Section 5.9). If data vary greatly, the confidence interval will be wider and more likely to overlap zero, implying non-significance. Greater SDs bring less power.

Standard of proof demanded (α)   A formal calculation of power technically needs to take into account the standard of proof being required for a declaration of significance. The usual criterion is that the 95 per cent confidence interval excludes a zero effect ($\alpha = 0.05$). If an experiment was designed to achieve a higher standards of proof (e.g. $\alpha = 0.02$), a 98 per cent CI will have to be used and this will be wider than the standard 95 per cent CI. The wider interval is then more likely to cross the zero line and so power will be lower. So, requiring a lower risk of a false positive (reducing alpha) will lead to less power.

The alpha value was included in the previous discussion, simply for the sake of completeness, but from this point on, we will ignore the question of standards of proof and simply assume that the normal standard is used (i.e. $\alpha = 0.05$; a 95 per cent CI is used or significance accepted if $P < 0.05$). Figure 8.3 shows the inputs into a formal calculation of the power of an experiment and the effects they would have.

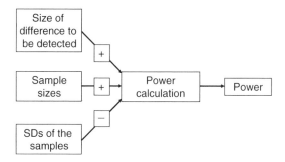

Figure 8.3 Calculation of the power of an experiment that will be analysed by a two-sample *t*-test

8.3 Calculating necessary sample size

Main factors affecting the power of a study

- The greater the sample size, the greater the power.

- The greater the experimental effect that we are trying to detect, the greater the power.

- The greater the variability in the data, the less the power.

8.3.1 The need for rational planning

In day-to-day practical experimentation, sample sizes probably owe more to tradition than logic. PhD students use five rats not on the basis of any rational calculation but simply because their supervisor always used five (and they in turn used five because their supervisors used five and so on *ad infinitum*.) There is now increasing recognition that hereditary malpractice ought to be replaced by soundly based optimization.

It is a sin to perform an experiment that is either too small or too large. Experiments that are excessively large are obviously a waste of resources. An answer could have been arrived at with less expenditure of time, effort and cash. If animals or humans were the subjects of the experiment, then there is also the ethical issue of unnecessary inconvenience or suffering. Experiments that are too small are perhaps even worse. If numbers are inadequate then the statistical analysis will almost certainly produce a non-significant result and we will be none the wiser. An effect may yet be present, but our pathetic little experiment could never have detected it. In that case all the expense and patient inconvenience were completely wasted. It is therefore important to plan the sizes of samples so they are big enough but not too big. Reviews of past literature suggest that, while examples of both under- and over-powered experiments exist, much the commonest problem is under-powering.

8.3.2   Factors influencing necessary sample size

The road to proper sample size planning begins here. In the same way that we can re-arrange an algebraic equation, we can also re-arrange one of our block diagrams. If we take Figure 8.3 which shows the factors that influence power, we can re-arrange it (Figure 8.4) to show the factors that influence necessary sample size.

The logic of these pluses and minuses is:

- *Size of experimental effect to be detectable* – large experimental effects are relatively easy to detect and small sample sizes will suffice, but smaller effects require larger sample sizes. The relationship is negative.

- *Standard deviation* – greater variability in the response will make it harder to detect an effect and so we will need larger sample sizes – a positive relationship.

- *Power required* – power increases with sample size, so if we want more power we will need larger samples – another positive relationship.

Figure 8.4 implies that, if we want to be able to calculate necessary sample size, we will need to supply values for each of the factors on the left of the diagram. At this point it would be useful to make a few additional comments about these three factors

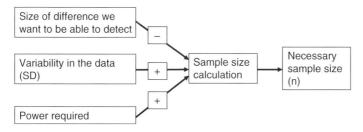

Figure 8.4 Calculation of necessary sample size for an experiment that will be analysed by a two-sample *t*-test

> ## ⌾ Main factors affecting necessary sample size
>
> • Size of difference to be detected.
>
> • Standard deviations in the samples.
>
> • Power to be achieved.

8.3.3   Size of experimental effect we want to be able to detect

The necessary sample size will be governed by the smallest difference we want to be able to detect. The latter is not based on statistical considerations. It can only be defined by somebody with expertise in the particular field. They should be able to say what sort of size of effect needs to be detectable.

There is always a temptation to be a super-perfectionist and insist that, if there is even the slightest difference, you want to know about it. However, if you set the detection limit to an excessively low value, the necessary sample size will probably escalate to something unmanageable! We have to accept that we cannot detect infinitesimally small effects and we must draw the limit at some reasonable point.

It is useful to consider 'What is the smallest experimental effect that would be of *practical* significance?' It is pointless trying to detect any effect much smaller than this figure. If we do try to detect a smaller effect, our experiment will be unnecessarily large and the extra cost and effort will merely enable us to detect effects that are too small to matter anyway! However, it is also important not to stray in the opposite direction. If we set the detection limit too high, this may yield a satisfyingly small sample size, but our experiment will now be too insensitive and may fail to detect a difference that is large enough to be of real practical significance.

> ## ⌾ Size of effect to be detected
>
> The figure we choose for the smallest difference we want to be able to detect should match the smallest effect that would be of real practical significance.
> No bigger. No smaller.

8.3.4   The SD among individual responses to the treatment

When a statistician who has been asked to plan the size of an experiment demands to know what the SD is going to be, the response is often quite shirty. 'How the devil would I know – I have not done the experiment yet' is not untypical. The objection is theoretically valid, but in practice rarely a real problem. There are several obvious solutions which include:

- Look in the literature for other experiments measuring the same endpoint and see how variable other people found it to be.

- Conduct a pilot experiment to estimate the SD and then plan the main experiment.

- Start the experiment and take a peek after the first few cases; use these to estimate the SD and then work out how big the experiment needs to be.

8.3.5 How powerful we want our experiment to be

Like the detection limit, this is also something that cannot be calculated statistically. It really depends upon the resources available and how critical the experiment is. It is usual to aim for a power somewhere between 80 and 95 per cent. Always remember that, if we go for greater power, a greater sample size will be required. If resources are plentiful and the experiment is critical then it might be perfectly reasonable to plan to achieve 95 per cent power. If data are either very difficult or expensive to generate then, you might be forced to settle for 80 per cent power.

8.3.6 An example – the theophylline clearance experiment

To calculate an appropriate sample size for the rifampicin/theophylline experiment, we need to establish suitable values for the three inputs to the power calculation.

Minimum effect to be detectable   We talk to some 'experts' and they decide that, if theophylline clearance is changed to an extent of ±20 per cent, they want to know about it. (The implication is that, if some smaller difference were present, but our experiment failed to detect it, it would be considered no big deal.) A typical text-book mean clearance for theophylline (under normal circumstances) is 0.67 ml/min/kg. Therefore, a 20 per cent change would equate to an increase or decrease of about 0.13 ml/min/kg.

Standard deviation among theophylline clearances   A review of the literature concerning the clearance of theophylline gave conflicting results, but a 'guesstimate' of SD = ±0.25 ml/min/kg was agreed upon.

Power to be achieved   Data for an experiment of this type are likely to be acquired quite slowly and will be expensive to obtain, so we are unlikely to want to try for a very high power such as 90 or 95 per cent. Furthermore, on ethical grounds, we do not want to expose unnecessarily large numbers of subjects to this dubious experiment, so we settle for 80 per cent power.

8.3.7   Using a statistical package to calculate necessary sample size

You may need to shop around for a statistics package that does calculations of necessary sample size. SPSS does not have this functionality as part of its standard package – you need access to an add-on (SamplePower[R]). Minitab is the winner in this regard – it does include suitable calculations for all simple experimental designs. Whatever package you end up using, you will have to provide values for the three inputs shown in Figure 8.4. Generic output is shown in Table 8.2.

   The number calculated is the number per group, so 120 subjects would have to be recruited and then divided into control and treated groups. It is obviously only possible to use exact whole numbers of subjects – fractional patients are impossible (unless some terrible accident has occurred). Generally, no exact number of subjects will provide precisely 80 per cent power, so your package should report the smallest whole number that will provide at least that much power. If your package reports a fractional number, then in order to provide at least adequate power, it should always be rounded up to the nearest integer – we do not round to the nearest integer if that would mean rounding downwards. The package also reports the actual power that will be achieved having rounded the number of subjects upwards.

8.3.8   Was our experiment big enough?

In our real experiment we used only 15 subjects per group, not 60, and yet, despite this, we got a clearly significant result. The main reason for this is that the sample size of 60 was calculated as being adequate to reveal a change of 0.13 ml/min/kg, whereas the actual difference found was almost 0.3 ml/min/kg. Because the real effect was so large, it was easy to detect and our small experiment proved adequate (more by good luck than good management).

   Notice that this still does not justify conducting such a limited experiment. If the difference had been (say) 0.2 ml/min/kg, that would been big enough for us to need to know about it, but our experiment would almost certainly have failed to detect it.

Table 8.2 Generic output for calculation of necessary sample size for the rifampicin/theophylline experiment

Sample size for two-sample *t*-test:

Assumed SD = 0.25
Difference to detect = 0.13
Power required = 0.8

Sample size = 60
Power achieved = 0.806

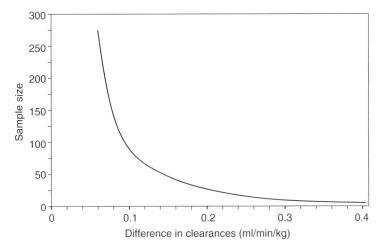

Figure 8.5 Necessary sample size when varying the size of difference to be detected (SD = 0.25 ml/min/kg and power = 80 per cent)

8.3.9 Sensitivity of necessary sample size to the three controlling factors

So far we have identified which factors influence necessary sample size. In the rest of this chapter we will see how great an effect each of these factors has.

Varying the minimum difference in clearance to be detectable In our sample size calculation, the minimum effect to be detectable was set at a change of 0.13 ml/min/ kg. What would happen if we varied this detection limit while maintaining everything else constant? Figure 8.5 shows the results. We already anticipated that necessary sample size would increase if we tried to detect small changes, but this figure shows that the relationship is an extremely sensitive one. In fact the necessary sample size depends approximately on the square of the detection limit. So if we tried to make the experiment 10 times more sensitive (i.e. reduce the detection limit by a factor of 10), the necessary sample size would increase 100 fold!

This serves to emphasize how important it is not to be overly ambitious. Any attempt to detect experimental effects that are trivially small could lead to astronomically large numbers.

Varying the standard deviation among theophylline clearances We can do a similar exercise, varying the assumed standard deviation among the clearances, while holding everything else constant. Figure 8.6 shows the results.

SD also has a powerful effect upon necessary sample size. This is also approximately a square relationship with sample size depending on the square of the SD. Therefore, if we could halve the variability in our data, the sample size would fall to about a quarter.

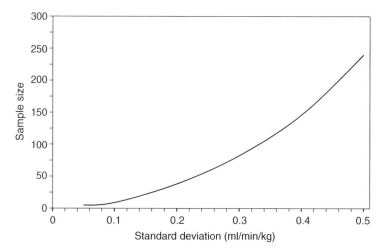

Figure 8.6 Necessary sample size when varying the SD for the samples (difference to be detectable = 0.13 ml/min/kg and power = 80 per cent)

It does therefore follow that it is very important to reduce the SD as much as possible. Theophylline clearances are intrinsically variable and there is nothing we can do about that. However, random measurement errors may be inflating the SD and we should certainly be attempting to eradicate all unnecessary sources of variability.

Varying the planned power of the study   Finally, we can vary the planned power for the study, while holding everything else constant. Figure 8.7 shows the results. As we anticipated, achieving increased power will require greater sample sizes. However,

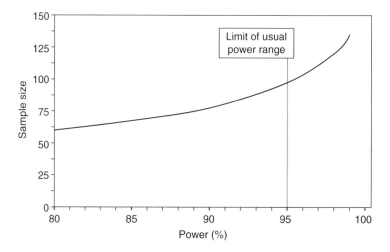

Figure 8.7 Necessary sample size when varying the planned power (difference to be detectable = 0.13 ml/min/kg and SD = 0.25 ml/min/kg)

the effect is quite modest. Within the commonly used range of power from 80 to 95 per cent, necessary sample size does not vary greatly. If we were to try to raise the power beyond 95 per cent, then sample sizes would start to increase uncomfortably, but it would be unusual to attempt to achieve such high power figures.

⚷ Factors influencing necessary sample size

Necessary sample size shows the following pattern of dependencies:

- highly sensitive to minimum effect to be detected;

- highly sensitive to the standard deviations within the samples;

- modestly sensitive to the planned power of the experiment.

8.4 Chapter summary

If we fail to detect a difference that truly is present, this constitutes a false negative or type II error. If a difference of a stated size is present, 'beta' is the risk that we will fail to detect it. Conversely, 'power' is the probability that we will detect it.

The main factors affecting power are:

- The greater the sample size, the greater the power.

- The greater the size of the difference that we are trying to detect, the greater the power.

- The greater the variability in the data, the less the power.

The design of all experiments should involve a rational calculation of how large the samples need to be. For an experiment that will be analysed by a two-sample t-test, the main influences upon necessary sample size are:

- Increasing the size of the difference that we want to be able to detect dramatically decreases sample sizes.

- Increasing the variability of the data dramatically increase sample sizes.

- Increasing the planned power of the experiment moderately increases sample sizes.

When calculating sample sizes, the figure for the smallest difference to be detectable should generally match the smallest difference that would be of practical significance.

9
The two-sample *t*-test (4). Statistical significance, practical significance and equivalence

This chapter will ...

- Show that a statistically significant difference is not synonymous with a practically significant difference

- Introduce equivalence limits and the equivalence zone

- Explain how to test for a practically significant difference between two measured outcomes

- Explain how to test for equivalence (i.e. show that two measured outcomes do not differ to an extent that is of practical significance)

- Explain how to test for non-inferiority (i.e. show that one product or process is at least as good as another)

Essential Statistics for the Pharmaceutical Sciences   Philip Rowe
© 2007 John Wiley & Sons, Ltd   ISBN 9780 470 03470 5 (HB)   ISBN 9780 470 03468 2 (PB)

9.1 Practical significance – is the difference big enough to matter?

Figure 6.9 showed the interplay between various factors in the outcome of a two-sample t-test. Two of these factors were the extent of the difference observed and the sample sizes. It is perfectly possible for a study to produce a statistically significant outcome even where the difference is very small, so long as the sample size is correspondingly large. In principal, there is no lower limit to the size of experimental effect that could be detected, if we were prepared to perform a big enough experiment. However, this can cause problems, as the next example demonstrates.

9.1.1 Detection of a trivially small effect upon haemoglobin levels

We want to check whether a widely used antidepressant might be having an effect upon haemoglobin levels (possibly by interfering with vitamin absorption). We have already accumulated a mass of basic clinical data from routine monitoring of patients taking various antidepressants. We simply ask the IT department to extract haemoglobin data for at least 200 patients taking the suspect medicine and from another 200 (plus) taking any anti-depressant other than the one that is suspect. These later will be our controls.

The data set is too large to reproduce here, but is available from the web site. The summary descriptive data is:

Controls: $n = 220$ mean haemoglobin $= 157.61 \pm 11.85$ g/l ($\pm$SD)
Suspect drug: $n = 235$ mean haemoglobin $= 155.10 \pm 12.19$ g/l ($\pm$SD)

There is some evidence of lower haemoglobin levels.

Subjecting this data to a two-sample t-test, we find that the point estimate for the difference between mean haemoglobin levels (expressed as suspect drug – control) is -2.51 g/l with a 95 per cent confidence interval of -0.294 to -4.728 g/l. As zero is excluded from the interval, there is significant evidence of a difference in haemoglobin levels.

The danger is that word 'significant'. For the uninitiated there will be a temptation to interpret 'significant' as indicating a difference big enough to be of practical importance. However, statistical significance is only an indication of whether or not there is a change, and tells us nothing about how big any difference might be. If we want to know whether the effect is big enough to matter, we need to look at the actual size of the change and compare this to what is known about the clinical significance of variations in haemoglobin levels.

⚖ Statistical and practical significance

Statistical significance – is there a difference?
Practical significance – is there a difference big enough to matter?

9.1.2 'Equivalence limits' and 'zone of equivalence'

As a first step towards a formal test of practical significance, we need to establish just how large any change would need to be for it to have practical consequences. This decision is not based on any statistical considerations – it depends upon the judgement of an expert in the particular field.

Experts suggest that we can be confident that any change of less than 6 g/l will have no practical consequences. This allows us to establish lower and upper 'equivalence limits' at −6 and +6 g/l. For the purposes of this discussion, we will assume that these patients tend to be somewhat anaemic, so a reduction of greater than 6 g/l would be detrimental and a similar sized increase would be beneficial. Between these possibilities, there is a 'zone of equivalence' (we are confident the patient will be neither better nor worse).

⚍ Equivalence limits

By how much would the parameter in question need to change before there was a realistic possibility of practical consequences? They are not calculated by any statistical procedure; they are based upon expert opinion.

We could then present the results of our haemoglobin experiment as a nice, intuitive diagram (Figure 9.1). Notice that the horizontal axis is the difference in haemoglobin levels in the two groups. The whole of the 95 per cent CI for the difference arising from use of the suspect drug lies within the zone of equivalence. Even looking at the greatest effect the suspect drug might realistically have (a change of 4.7 g/l), this is still too small to be of any consequence.

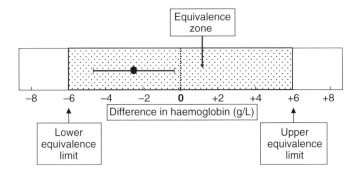

Figure 9.1 The confidence interval for the difference in haemoglobin levels in relation to the equivalence zone

---

🔑 Haemoglobin levels

- The results are *statistically* significant. The 95 per cent CI excludes zero, so there is evidence of a difference between the two groups.

- The results are not *practically* significant. The difference is too small.

9.1.3   General interpretation of practical significance

The general way in which we would determine the practical significance of a change in haemoglobin levels is summarized in Figure 9.2, assuming that decreases in haemoglobin would be detrimental and increases beneficial.

The first three cases are unambiguous. (a) is detrimental and definitely of practical significance. We are pretty confident that even the minimum effect (a reduction of 7.5 g/l) is large enough to cause practical harm. (b) definitely has no practical significance; the whole CI is within the equivalence zone. (c) is beneficial and definitely of practical significance. The most pessimistic view would be that there is an increase of 7 g/l, which is still enough to be useful.

In the remaining cases, the CI crosses between zones and the result is ambiguous. We are limited as to what conclusions can be drawn and judgement has to be exercised. The only definite thing we can say in (d) is that it is not doing any good, since none of the 95 per cent CI extends into the zone of practical benefit. Most of the CI is in the zone of practical detriment, so we would almost certainly want to avoid whatever caused this effect, even if it is not yet proven to be doing practical harm. (e) definitely does no practical harm, and may be beneficial. The CI is quite wide and a

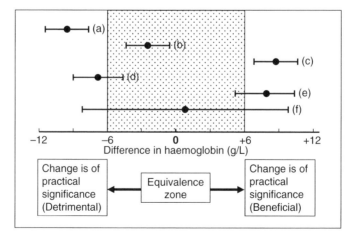

Figure 9.2   Determining the practical significance for differences in haemoglobin levels

larger experiment should narrow it, with reasonable prospects that it would then emerge as unambiguously beneficial. (f) is completely ambiguous. We can say nothing definite. The treatment could be beneficial, harmful or have no noticeable effect. The experiment appears to have been of very low power.

⚓ Practical significance

To demonstrate that a treatment produces an effect great enough to be of practical significance, we must show that the 95 per cent CI for the size of the treatment effect lies entirely to one side of the equivalence zone.

9.1.4 Unequal sample sizes

In the previous example, the two samples differed slightly in size. This does not invalidate the *t*-test; The calculation of the test can incorporate such inequalities without difficulty. The only reason we normally use balanced designs (equal numbers in both groups) is that, for any total number of observations, statistical power is greatest if they are split equally. In this case the imbalance is so small that any loss of power will be trivial. However, if imbalance leads to one of the groups being quite small, the loss of power may make the whole exercise futile.

⚓ Balanced samples

To maintain statistical power, try to avoid major imbalances between the sizes of the two samples being compared.

9.2 Equivalence testing

Traditional statistical testing tends to focus on attempts to demonstrate that a measured value changes according to what treatment is used. This is called 'difference testing'. However, there are occasions when we want to show that a measured value does not change. This, we would call 'equivalence testing'.

Typical cases where we might wish to demonstrate equivalence include:

- Changing a pharmaceutical formulation of a drug. The important factor might be that the new preparation delivers the same amount of drug as the old one. We want patients to be able to switch from the old to the new preparation without their effective dose changing.

- Replacing an existing analytical method with one that is newer and simpler. We would like to show that, if a sample were analysed by both methods, we would get the same answer.

There is a problem, however – it is impossible to demonstrate that there is absolutely no difference between two treatments or procedures. Take the first of the cases above – the two drug preparations. Could we ever demonstrate that they deliver exactly the same amount of active material? The answer must be 'no'. Any experiment we conduct will be finite in size and can therefore only detect differences down to a certain size. However large an experiment we conduct, there could always be some tiny difference just too small for the current experiment to detect. It is therefore impossible to demonstrate that two preparations behave absolutely identically. Similarly, we could never show that two analytical methods produce exactly the same answers.

Since we cannot demonstrate exact equality, we turn instead to practical equivalence. We try to demonstrate that any possible difference between two outcome is too small to be of practical significance.

Equivalence testing is conducted in three stages:

1. Determine an equivalence zone, based on expert knowledge of the likely effect of a change of any given size.

2. Determine the 95 per cent CI for the difference between the two products/ methods or whatever else is being tested.

3. Check to see if the whole of the 95 per cent CI for any difference fits entirely within the equivalence zone. If it does, then we have a positive demonstration of practical equivalence. If either end of the interval extends beyond the equivalence zone, then equivalence cannot be assured.

⚷ Equivalence testing

Equivalence testing is designed to show that there are no differences big enough to be worth worrying about. To demonstrate equivalence, the whole of the 95 per cent CI for the size of any difference should lie entirely within the equivalence zone.

9.2.1 An example of equivalence testing – comparing two propranolol formulations

Propranolol is a drug used to reduce blood pressure. It is known that only a limited proportion (about a third) of the dose swallowed actually survives intact and gets into the patient's blood system. When changing the formulation of such a drug, one

Table 9.1 Areas under the curve (AUCs) for old and new formulations of propranolol

AUCs for old preparation (µg·h/l)				AUCs for new preparation (µg·h/l)			
555	493	569	500	505	746	431	556
495	272	418	365	595	525	362	497
736	592	673	667	549	665	585	675
699	379	544	623	679	490	727	566
377	734	604	552	559	645	524	564
573	709	649	573	604	593	559	684
692	752	527	681	474	596	403	674
270	756	571	688	515	678	577	532
596	690	633	196	547	432	613	532
508	457	475	531	546	581	434	431
582	369	472	461	611	501	554	570
668	500	495	552	601	506	525	550
538	425	659	497	648	621	608	655
600	689	603	493	412	518	729	
686	697	588	522	483	537	586	
Mean = 557.8 ± 124.6 µg·h/l				Mean = 563.2 ± 84.7 µg·h/l			

would want to be assured that the proportion being successfully absorbed did not suddenly change. The best marker of absorption is the so-called AUC, i.e. the area under the curve for the graph of blood concentration vs time. This is measured in units of µg·h/l. Table 9.1 shows the AUC values when a series of individuals take either the old or the new preparations.

It is decided that the new and old preparations are unlikely to show any clinically significant difference in effectiveness if we can be assured that their AUCs do not differ by more than 10 per cent. Since the old preparation produced a mean AUC of 556 µg·h/l, and 10 per cent of this is approximately 55 µg·h/l, the equivalence zone is set to cover a mean change of −55 to +55 µg·h/l.

Next we generate a confidence interval by carrying out a two-sample *t*-test. The point estimate for the difference (defined as AUCnew − AUCold) is 5.4 µg·h/l with a 95 per cent confidence interval for the difference between the two preparations of −33.6 to +44.3 µg·h/l.

This is shown in Figure 9.3 along with the equivalence zone.

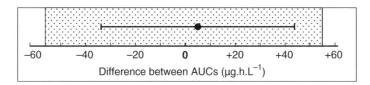

Figure 9.3 The 95 per cent CI for difference between AUCs of two propranolol formulations (new − old). The shaded area is the equivalence zone

The whole of the 95 per cent CI fits within the equivalence zone. Therefore, we have positively demonstrated that, if there is any difference between the two preparations, it is too small to be of practical consequence. The two formulations have been demonstrated to be effectively equivalent.

9.2.2 Difference vs equivalence testing. Same test – different interpretations

Notice that difference and equivalence testing use exactly the same statistical calculation. In both cases, a two-sample *t*-test is used to generate a 95 per cent CI for difference. It is the interpretation that differs.

When testing for

- statistically significant difference – is zero excluded from the CI?

- practically significant difference – is the whole of the CI to one side of the equivalence zone?

- equivalence – is the whole of the CI within the equivalence zone?

9.2.3 Caution – comparing analytical methods

Equivalence testing (as described) would form a necessary part of any demonstration that two analytical methods were interchangeable, but it would not be sufficient alone. If you need to tackle this problem, consult a specialized text.

9.2.4 How *not* to test for equivalence

A common misapplication of statistics is to test for equivalence by performing a test for difference, obtaining a non-significant result and then claiming that, because

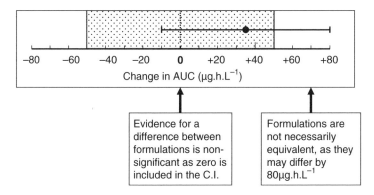

Figure 9.4 Results that should *not* be claimed as providing evidence of equivalence

there is no evidence of any difference, the two things must be equivalent. The fallacy of this approach is immediately visible if we think about a possible result for our comparison of propranolol formulations. Figure 9.4 shows a case where the result of a test for difference would be declared statistically non-significant, since a zero difference is included within the 95 per cent CI However, the formulations are not necessarily equivalent, since there is a real possibility that the new formulation may be producing values up to 80 µg.h/l greater than the old.

  ## Make that embarrassing difference disappear

If your target journal sends your paper to a statistically savvy reviewer, you will not get away with this one, but do not worry – many of them do not.

Your new treatment or analytical method (or whatever) is supposed to produce the same results as the old one, but the wretched thing obviously does not. Do not despair, just follow these simple instructions:

- set up a comparison of the new vs the old using a small sample size that you know to be suitably underpowered;

- carry out a statistical test for difference and get a non-significant result;

- swear blind that, as you did not show a difference, the new system must produce the same results as the old one;

- should this fail, simply repeat with a smaller and smaller sample size, until you force the difference to stop being statistically significant.

 ## 'Absence of evidence is not evidence of absence'

The failure to find a difference, does not necessarily imply that none exists. Maybe you did not look very hard.

9.3 Non-inferiority testing

9.3.1 Change in dialysis method

With equivalence testing there are two possibilities that we need to dispose of – the possibilities that the difference between outcomes might be either (a) greater than some upper limit or (b) less than a lower limit. The propranolol tablets provide an example of this. It would be potentially dangerous for the patient if the amount of drug absorbed suddenly increased or decreased, and we have to exclude both possibilities. However, there are many cases where our only worry is that a particular value might (say) decrease. In that case, presumably an increase in the value would be perfectly acceptable (we would either welcome an increase or at least be neutral about it). The question now being asked is 'is the new product/method, etc., at least as good as the old one?' This is referred to as 'non-inferiority testing'.

⌐O At least as good as . . .

Non-inferiority testing is used to see whether a product/process is at least as good as some alternative.

Take, as an example, the use of dialysis in renally compromised patients. We have an established method, but want to evaluate a possible alternative which would be simpler, if it is clinically acceptable. A key endpoint is plasma urea concentration. If changing the dialysis method were to lead to an increase in urea levels, this would be unacceptable. On the other hand, a decrease in urea levels would be a bonus, but is not essential. Clinical judgement is that a difference in urea levels of ±1 mM is the smallest change likely to cause a noticeable effect in the patient.

A series of possible outcomes from a comparison of the two methods is shown in Figure 9.5. In this case, the shaded area is not an equivalence zone as this is no longer relevant. What is now shown is the 'failure zone'. Differences in this zone would be indicative of a rise in urea concentrations too great to be acceptable.

One-tailed 95 per cent confidence limits have been calculated (as described in Section 5.8). The confidence limit calculated is always that which indicates the most

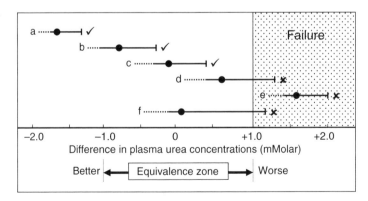

Figure 9.5 Interpretation of non-inferiority testing. Comparison of new dialysis method with old. Difference in plasma urea concentration (mM)

pessimistic view. We then check whether this worst possible value would represent a deterioration of a magnitude that would actually matter.

In the current case, we calculate the upper confidence limit as this indicates the worst credible interpretation of the data. Then, the condition for acceptance of the new treatment is that this upper limit does not enter the failure zone starting at +1 mM. As the decision is based solely on this upper limit, a lower limit would have served no useful purpose and was not calculated.

Notice the difference. For equivalence testing we have to show that any change lies between an upper and a lower limit, but with non-inferiority testing we only have to show that there is no change beyond a single (upper or lower) limit.

The top three cases (a–c) would all pass a test of non-inferiority, as they preclude an increase in plasma urea great enough to cause any appreciable deterioration in patients' conditions. With the remaining three cases, however, we could not, at this stage, claim to have demonstrated non-inferiority. In all three cases a deterioration large enough to be of concern remains a possibility. Treatment (e) looks like a pretty hopeless case and could probably be discounted as a candidate. The other two – (d) and (f) – might be acceptable, but larger trials would be required in order to narrow the confidence intervals and then either (or both) of them might be established as non-inferior.

> ## ⊸○ Non-inferiority testing
>
> Can we demonstrate that the new product/procedure is at least as good as that with which it is being compared? We must be able to show that the most pessimistic one-sided confidence limit excludes any adverse difference large enough to be of practical significance.

9.4 *P* values are less informative and can be positively misleading

All of the above procedures – demonstration that a change is large enough to be of practical significance or demonstration of equivalence or non-inferiority – are entirely dependent upon the use of the 95 per cent CI for the size of the treatment effect. *P* values would be pointless (unless we wanted to cheat!).

However, *P* values are not only less informative than the 95 per cent CI; they can even be downright misleading, if taken in isolation. Table 9.2 gives the results of two trials of candidate antipyretic drugs (A and B). A beneficial effect would consist of a reduction in temperature and clinical judgement is that a reduction of at least 0.5°C would be required for patients to feel any benefit. It is also assumed that a rise of 0.5°C would be detrimental.

Table 9.2 Results of two trials of potential antipyretics

Drug	Sample sizes	Difference between mean temperatures (°C)	P
A	200	−0.247	0.009 Significant
B	15	−0.537	0.074 Non-significant

On the basis of the *P* values alone, drug A appears to be worth further development as it is produces a statistically significant effect, whereas there is no significant evidence that B produces any effect and the temptation would be to drop the latter. However, in Figure 9.6 we assess the same data using the 95 per cent CIs and combine these with our assumption that a practically significant temperature change would have to be of at least 0.5°C. This suggests exactly the opposite conclusion. Drug A does produce an effect, but this is positively demonstrated to be too small to be of any clinical value. With B, the experiment is very small and the confidence interval correspondingly wide. Consequently, the interval overlaps zero and the result is not statistically significant, however a large part of the confidence interval is in the area that would be of practical benefit. There is therefore still a reasonable chance that B may produce an effect, and furthermore this may be big enough to be useful. If we are going to expend money/effort on further development of either of these candidates, B is the better bet, not A.

The implementation of the two-sample *t*-test offered in Excel is very unfortunate as it provides a *P* value but no confidence interval for the difference.

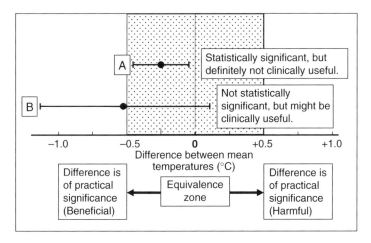

Figure 9.6 Correct interpretation of possible antipyretic preparations A and B

> **⚷ The superiority of the 95 per cent CI**
>
> To demonstrate practical superiority, equivalence or non-inferiority, we must inspect the 95 per cent confidence interval for the difference between mean values. The P value is completely irrelevant to all these questions and is potentially misleading.

9.5 Setting equivalence limits prior to experimentation

Equivalence limits should be set before experimental work begins. It is very difficult to decide objectively where equivalence limits should be placed if you already know the experimental results and what the consequence would be of placing the limits at any particular level.

For the sake of your own credibility it is also very useful if you can register the decision with some independent party, prior to experimentation. That way, everybody else can be assured that the placing of the limits has not been inappropriately influenced.

> **Make the limits do the work**
>
> If you push this one too far, it will stand out like a sore thumb, but within reason, you might get away with it.
>
> Your new product/method . . .
>
> - worked, but not very well; or
>
> - is obviously different from the old one, when it should have been the same; or
>
> - is annoyingly inferior to the old one.
>
> However, there is still the question of where we are going to put those pesky equivalence limits. In the first case, we will adjust them nice and close to zero, then even our pathetic effort will cause a 'practically significant' difference. For the latter two, we will invent some reason to set them generously wide and hey presto, we are 'equivalent' or 'non-inferior'.
>
> What you need is a journal that still has not twigged that they should be getting authors to declare these things in advance – i.e. pretty well any of them.

9.6 Chapter summary

A demonstration of statistical significance provides evidence that the treatment being investigated does make a difference, but it tells us nothing about whether that effect is large enough to be of practical significance. Large experiments/trials are liable to detect trivially small effects as being statistically significant.

The upper 'equivalence limit' is set to a value such that an increase to any lesser value would be of no practical consequence. Similarly, a lower equivalence limit defines the smallest decrease that would of practical relevance. Establishing the numerical value of these limits is based solely upon expert opinion. The range of values between the two equivalence limits is the 'equivalence zone'.

Demonstrating that a difference is of practical significance   To demonstrate that a treatment produces a change that is of practical significance, we need to show that the 95 per cent CI for the size of the difference lies entirely to one side of the equivalence zone.

Demonstrating equivalence   It is impossible to demonstrate that there is absolutely no difference between two procedures or treatments, but we may be able to show that there is no difference large enough to matter ('equivalence testing'). We need to demonstrate that the whole of the 95 per cent CI for the size of any difference lies within the equivalence zone. A non-significant result arising from a test for difference is not an adequate demonstration of equivalence.

Demonstrating non-inferiority   To demonstrate that a procedure or treatment is at least as good as an alternative (without needing to show that it is any better) requires 'non-inferiority' testing. We calculate a one-sided 95 per cent confidence limit for the difference between the two treatments. The limit calculated is the one that indicates the greatest credible deterioration associated with the new procedure. If this limit precludes any realistic possibility of a deterioration large enough to matter, we may claim evidence of non-inferiority.

Equivalence limits should always be fixed prior to undertaking experimental work and if possible the selected values should be registered at the same early stage.

10

The two-sample *t*-test (5). One-sided testing

This chapter will . . .

- Introduce the use of one-sided tests where an experiment was designed to find out whether an end-point changes in a specified direction and describe the special form of null-hypothesis used in one-sided tests

- Describe the use of one-sided confidence intervals to test such null hypotheses

- Show that, in marginal cases, data may be non-significant when assessed by a two-sided test, and yet be significant with the one-sided version of the same test

- Review the age-old trick of switching from a two-sided to a one-sided test thereby converting disappointing non-significance to the much coveted significance

- Show that said trick is not acceptable because it raises the risk of a false positive to 10 per cent instead of the standard 5 per cent

- Set out the correct protocol for using one-sided tests

Essential Statistics for the Pharmaceutical Sciences   Philip Rowe
© 2007 John Wiley & Sons, Ltd   ISBN 9780 470 03470 5 (HB)   ISBN 9780 470 03468 2 (PB)

10.1 Looking for a change in a specified direction

Sometimes, we may want to use a *t*-test in a way that differs from our previous approach. Say, for example, we are considering the use of urinary acidification to hasten the clearance of amphetamine from patients who have overdosed. An initial trial in rabbits is used to test the general principal. One group of rabbits receives ammonium chloride to induce a lower urinary pH and another group acts as controls. All rabbits receive a test dose of radio-labelled drug, the clearance of which is studied over a few hours. In this case, the question posed should be 'is there an *increase* in clearance?' rather than the standard 'is there a *difference* in clearance?' The former constitutes a one-sided question.

It often perplexes people that they cannot simply consider how an experiment was performed in order to tell whether a one or a two-sided test should be used. The fact is that the decision depends upon what question the experiment was designed to answer. If the purpose was to look for any old change – use a two-sided test. If your only interest lay in checking for a change in a particular, specified direction, a one-sided test should be used.

⚷ One- and two-sided questions

Is there a *change* in clearance? The answer will be 'yes' if there is either a marked increase or a marked decrease. This is a *two-sided* question.

Is there an *increase* in clearance? The answer will only be 'yes' if there is a marked change in the specified direction. This is a *one-sided* question.

10.1.1 Null and alternative hypotheses for testing one-sided questions

If we are going to test a one-sided question, we need to modify our null and alternative hypotheses. For two-sided testing, the null hypothesis would be that there is no difference in clearance and the alternative would be that there is. For a one-sided test (looking for a greater clearance) we want our alternative hypothesis to be 'there is an *increase* in clearance'. The null hypothesis then has to cover all other possibilities – 'clearance is either unchanged or reduced'.

🔑 Hypotheses for a one-sided test looking for an increase in clearance

Null hypothesis – for a very large group (population), the mean clearance among actively treated rabbits is either equal to or less than that in controls.

Alternative hypothesis – for a very large group (population), the mean clearance among actively treated rabbits is greater than that in controls.

In Chapter 5, we saw that we can generate a one-sided 95 per cent confidence interval by calculating a 90 per cent confidence interval and then using just one limit and ignoring the other. We can then say that there is only a 5 per cent chance that the true mean value lies beyond the one limit that is being quoted. We do essentially the same to perform a one-sided test for increased clearance. The steps are:

1. Make a firm decision that we are only testing for evidence of an increase in clearance.

2. Calculate the mean clearance for both groups.

3. Generate a 90 per cent CI for the difference between these mean clearances.

4. Only quote the confidence limit that acts as a test of the null hypothesis (in this case the lower limit).

5. Check whether this lower confidence limit is above zero. If it is, we have evidence of increased clearance.

Figure 10.1 shows how we would interpret the various possible outcomes of a one-sided test for an increase.

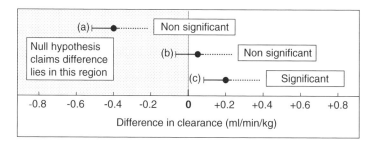

Figure 10.1 Interpretation of the confidence interval for the difference between mean clearances, when performing a one-sided test for evidence of an increase

The parts of the graph that correspond to the null hypothesis (no change or a decrease) are shown shaded in Figure 10.1. Only case (c) would be interpreted as a significant result, as it alone excludes all the territory claimed by the null hypothesis. With cases (a) and (b), a reduced or unchanged clearance is possible and the null hypothesis cannot be rejected. It might be thought that case (a) looks as if it means something significant, but the question being addressed is 'is there evidence of an *increase* in clearance?' and case (a) in no way supports any such notion.

Notice that, in this case, it is the lower limit of the CI that is used to make the decision – if it is above zero, the result is significant. If we had been testing for a reduction in clearance, we would have inspected the upper limit and the result would have been declared significant, if that was below zero.

⚿ Performing one-sided tests

*One-sided test for an **increase** in the measured value* – quote the lower confidence limit and declare the result significant if it is above zero (a reduced/unchanged value has been successfully excluded).

*One-sided test for a **decrease** in the measured value* – quote the upper confidence limit and declare the result significant if it is below zero (an increased/unchanged value has been successfully excluded).

10.2 Protection against false positives

With all statistical tests, one aim is to ensure that, where there is no real effect, we will make false positive claims on only 5 per cent of occasions. Consider what would happen if there was actually no effect on clearance and we carried out 20 trials, each analysed by a one-sided test (testing for an increase). Bearing in mind that the actual procedure is to calculate a 90 per cent CI, but then convert it to what is effectively a 95 per cent CI by ignoring one of its limits, we can predict the likely outcomes as in Figure 10.2:

- *Eighteen times out of 20, the 90 per cent confidence interval will span zero* – the lower limit is below zero, so the null hypothesis cannot be rejected. The result is correctly declared as non-significant.

- *One time in 20, the entire interval will be below zero* – the lower limit is again below zero and the result is correctly interpreted as non-significant.

- *One time in 20, the entire interval will be above zero* – the lower limit is now above zero and the result will be falsely interpreted as providing significant evidence of increased clearance.

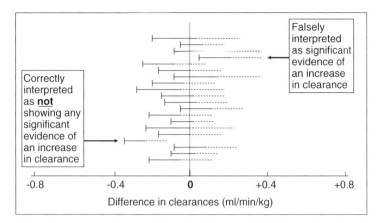

Figure 10.2 Twenty one-sided 95 per cent confidence intervals for change in clearance when there is no real treatment effect (one-sided tests for evidence of an increase)

Thus we have achieved our goal. If there is no real difference, there is only a 5 per cent chance that we will falsely declare significant evidence of an increase in clearance.

⚷ Protection from false positives

Where a treatment has no real effect, a properly conducted, one-sided test will expose us to the standard 5 per cent risk of a false positive conclusion that there is an effect in the direction tested for.

10.3 Temptation!

10.3.1 Data may be Significant with a one-sided test, even though it was non-significant with a two-sided test

Table 10.1 shows a set of results for an investigation of the effects of urinary acidification on the clearance of amphetamine. We could test this set of results using two different approaches:

- a one-sided test looking for increased clearance as discussed earlier;

- a normal two-sided test looking for any change in clearance.

The confidence limits for the difference are:

One-sided test (lower limit only)	$+0.021$
Two-sided test (lower and upper limits)	-0.031 to $+0.582$

Table 10.1 Clearance (ml/min/kg) of an amphetamine with and without urinary acidification

	Control	Acidification
	1.84	1.37
	1.19	0.25
	1.02	1.26
	0.71	1.87
	0.98	2.14
	1.27	1.42
	1.27	1.26
	0.68	0.97
	1.43	1.78
	1.55	1.54
	1.28	1.51
	1.03	1.98
	1.21	2.06
	1.57	1.22
	1.14	1.67
Mean	1.211	1.487
± SD	± 0.312	± 0.482

These are shown diagrammatically in Figure 10.3. For the one-sided test, the confidence limit began life as a part of a 90 per cent confidence interval, which is narrower than the 95 per cent CI used for the two-sided test. In this case, the difference in width just happens to make a critical difference – the two-sided test is not significant, but the one-sided test is.

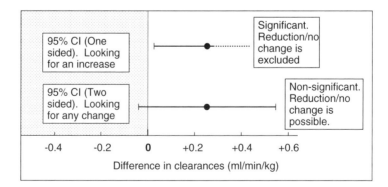

Figure 10.3 A one-sided test (for an increase) and a two-sided test (for any difference) in clearance

---

⚎ Significance with a one-sided, but not a two-sided test

In marginal cases, results that are not significant when tested with a two-sided test may just achieve statistical significance if re-tested with a one-sided test.

There are references above to both a significant and non-significant conclusion. However, if the question was whether there was an increase in clearance and there had been a prior decision to carry out a one-sided test, then the correct conclusion is that there is significant evidence of an increase. It should perhaps also be said that the results may be statistically significant, but the size of change is probably not of practical significance.

The P value for the one-sided test is 0.038, in line with our previous conclusion that it produced a significant result. The two-sided test would yield a P value exactly twice as large, i.e. 0.076 (non-significant).

10.3.2 Possible cheat

This obviously raises the possibility of abuse. If we initially performed the experiment intending to carry out a two-sided test and obtained a non-significant result, we might then be tempted to change to the one-sided test in order to force it to be significant.

10.3.3 Chances of a false positive would be raised to 10 per cent

The problem with such an approach is illustrated in Figure 10.4, in which we consider a case where there is no real experimental effect and we insist on looking at the results

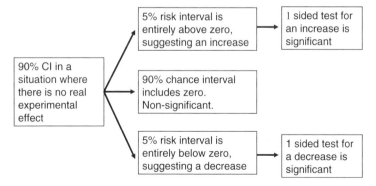

Figure 10.4 A 10 per cent chance of a false positive outcome if we abuse one-sided testing by choosing the direction of test after results are known

first and then performing a one-sided test in whatever direction suits our purposes. A 90 per cent confidence interval is initially calculated, so there is a 10 per cent likelihood that the interval will not include the true value of a zero change. This will be made up of a 5 per cent risk that it will suggest an increase and another 5 per cent that it will suggest a reduction. In this case, we have already seen the results and can guarantee that the one-sided test we carry out will be in the 'appropriate' direction to give a significant result. Therefore, in total, we now have a 10 per cent chance of a false positive.

⚊◉ Improper use of one-sided tests

If a one-sided test is improperly selected after the data has been seen, we raise the risk of a false positive from the stated level of 5 per cent to a real level of 10 per cent.

10.3.4 One-sided tests must be conducted to a strict protocol if they are to be credible

A properly conducted one-sided procedure would involve us committing ourselves to the direction of testing in advance. If we had committed ourselves to testing only for (say) an increase in clearance, then the 5 per cent of cases apparently showing a reduction in clearance (lowest branch in Figure 10.4) would not be declared significant and our false positive rate would remain where it should be – 5 per cent.

⚊◉ The fair way to perform one-sided tests

If a one-sided test is to be performed, the following steps must be taken *in the order shown*:

1. Decide that the test is to be one-sided and which direction of change will be tested for.

2. Perform the experiment.

3. Analyse the data according to the pre-specified plan.

Because the cheat outlined below is so easy to work, one-sided testing has fallen into considerable disrepute. That is a shame, because one-sided tests do have a perfectly respectable and useful role, if used appropriately. We can only hope that journal editors will, before too long, offer authors the opportunity to record our intentions in advance, to stop colleagues sniggering behind our backs when we use one-sided tests.

 Switch to a one-sided test after seeing the results

Even today, this is probably the best and most commonly used statistical fiddle. Powerful – undetectable – c'est magnifique!

You did the experiment and analysed the results by your usual two-sided test. The result fell just short of significance. There is a simple solution – guaranteed to work every time. Re-run the analysis, but change to a one-sided test, testing for a change in whatever direction you now know the results actually suggest. If P was originally anything between 0.05 and 0.1, this manoeuvre will exactly halve the P value and significance is assured.

Until scientific journals get their act together, and start insisting that authors register their intentions in advance, there is no way to detect this excellent fiddle. You just need some plausible reason why you 'always intended' to do a one-tailed test in this particular direction, and you are guaranteed to get away with it.

10.4 Using a computer package to carry out a one-sided test

For clarity, the test has been described in terms of generating a 90 per cent CI and using just one limit, but with most statistical packages the practical approach is to select an option for the direct performance of a one-sided test. You will also have to indicate the direction of change that is to be tested for. The programme will then generate a 95 per cent confidence limit (either upper or lower, as requested) and a P value should also be produced. Typical output is shown in Table 10.2.

Table 10.2 Generic output from a one-sided two-sample t-test for higher clearances with urinary acidification

Two-sample t-test (one-sided option selected)	
Mean (treated)	1.487
Mean (control)	1.211
Difference (treated – control)	+0.212
95% confidence limit for difference (lower)	+0.021
P	0.038

10.5   Should one-sided tests be used more commonly?

In statistics, two-sided testing is generally treated as the standard approach with one-sided methods seen as an alternative. While the author has never systematically surveyed research papers, one would suspect that a high proportion of experiments are in reality checking for change in a known direction. It is not very often that researchers actually say 'I want to see whether changing this factor causes some sort of change (maybe, an increase, maybe a decrease, who knows?)' In most cases he/she will not have chosen that factor randomly; it will have been selected because there was some reason to suspect that it would have an effect. If we have a likely mechanism in mind, it is also likely that one would anticipate change in a particular direction.

It is impossible to be sure, but there must be a suspicion that it is the general odour of abuse surrounding one-sided testing that inhibits researchers from using what is a perfectly legitimate and more powerful approach. If journals offered contributors the opportunity to register their intentions in advance, we could use one-sided tests without looking as if we are trying to pull a fast one.

10.6   Chapter summary

One-sided testing can be used where the purpose of the experiment is to test for changes in one particular direction. In the case of a one-sided test for an increased value, the null hypothesis is that the value is either unchanged or reduced and the alternative is that it is increased.

One-sided tests are conducted by generating the appropriate confidence limit for a one-sided 95 per cent CI (this may be achieved by calculating a 90 per cent confidence interval and discarding one of the limits). When testing for an increase, the lower confidence limit is used and vice versa.

If the confidence limit excludes the possibilities proposed by the null hypothesis, the outcome is statistically significant. With a properly conducted one-sided test, the risk of an accidental false positive when investigating a treatment that has no real effect is held at the usual 5 per cent.

Data may be non-significant with a two-sided test, and yet significant with a one-sided test. This can be abused to convert a non-significant finding to apparent significance. Such abuses raise the risk of false positives from 5 to 10 per cent.

One-sided tests should only be used if a firm decision had already been made to do so and the direction of change to be tested for had also been decided upon, before the data was generated. There may well be considerable under-use of one-sided tests because of difficulties in demonstrating that the decision to use these methods was indeed made at an appropriately early stage.

11

What does a statistically significant result really tell us?

This chapter will . . .

- Demonstrate that a statistically significant result does not lead to a fixed level of confidence that there really is a difference in outcomes between two treatments

- Suggest that significance tells us that we need to increase our level of confidence that there is a difference, but that what we end up believing depends upon the strength of the prior evidence

- Show that treatments for which there is already a sound basis of support can be accepted as virtually proven, given new, statistically significant evidence

- Suggest that intrinsically unlikely treatments should only be accepted if confirmed by several significant findings

11.1 Interpreting statistical significance

Just how strong is the evidence when we obtain a statistically significant result? It has already been emphasized on a number of occasions that it is not proof absolute. Even

Essential Statistics for the Pharmaceutical Sciences   Philip Rowe
© 2007 John Wiley & Sons, Ltd   ISBN 9780 470 03470 5 (HB)   ISBN 9780 470 03468 2 (PB)

when significance is demonstrated, there is still a residual possibility that we could have obtained unrepresentative and therefore misleading samples. However, it is not satisfactory simply to say that some doubt remains; people want to know how much doubt/certainty we are left with.

11.1.1 You cannot simply interpret a confidence interval as providing any set level of proof

There is a common misconception that, because methods like the two-sample t-test are based on 95 per cent confidence intervals, then 95 per cent of all significant results are true positives and 5 per cent are false. If only it were so simple! The following example will show that sadly it is not. We need to imagine two research workers. One works in early phase clinical trials and it is her job to test whether candidate drugs really do have pharmacological activity in humans. All the substances have already been extensively tested in other mammals and found to be active. Clearly there will be a few substances that are active in rats and dogs but not in humans, but in the great majority of cases they will also work in us. We will also consider somebody looking for pharmacological activity among traditional herbal remedies for which there is no existing scientific evidence of activity. Among such materials there will be a proportion that is effective, but it will probably be a small minority. Let us assume the following:

- Among the substances proven to be effective in other mammals, 90 per cent are also genuinely effective in humans.

- Among the traditional remedies, 10 per cent are genuinely effective in humans.

- Both researchers carry out statistical testing using the usual standard of significance (95 per cent CIs).

- Both design their experiments to achieve 90 per cent power.

- All products are either completely inactive or they have a level of activity that exactly matches the figure used to plan experimental size.

In Figure 11.1, 200 compounds that have already shown activity in other species should include 90 per cent (180) that are truly active in humans and 10 per cent (20) that lack activity. When the 180 genuinely active molecules are subjected to experiments with 90 per cent power, 162 trials will successfully detect that activity but 18 will fail to do so. Among the 20 inactive compounds, there will be the usual 5 per cent rate of false positives (one case). There are thus a total of 163 positive findings of which only one is false.

Figure 11.2 does the same analysis for 200 traditional herbal remedies. The big difference is that there are now 180 inactive substances which throw up a far greater

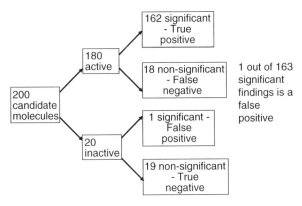

Figure 11.1 Investigating products where there is already a high level of evidence of activity

number (nine) of false positives. Among the total of 27 positive findings, fully one-third are false positives.

Therefore, there is no simple answer to the question as to how much assurance a significant result actually provides. It depends upon what is usually referred to as the 'prior evidence'. With the situation depicted in Figure 11.1, any given candidate molecule is already known to have a high prior likelihood of activity and obtaining a significant result very nearly guarantees true activity (one chance in 163 of an error). However with the traditional remedies, even if a particular material does come up with a significant result, we still need to be very cautious – there remains a one-third chance that it is not truly active.

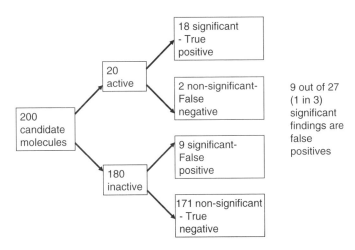

Figure 11.2 Investigating products where activity is unlikely

---

🔑 Look at all the previously available evidence as well as today's *P* value

Two experiments may produce exactly the same *P* value, but that does not mean that they necessarily lead to the same level of certainty that there is a true difference in outcome.

- If previous evidence (or basic scientific principles) already suggests a difference is very likely, a significant result will give a high level of confidence that there is a true difference.

- If prior information suggests that a real difference is unlikely, even a significant result will still leave considerable doubt.

11.1.2   Statistical results tell us how to modify our existing beliefs

The results of statistical tests are best interpreted in terms of how much they change our view rather than expecting them to tell us what we should end up believing. Figure 11.3 illustrates the idea. With a molecule already known to be active in other mammals, we start out knowing that it is likely to be active in humans. A significant finding then boosts our faith in it to something approaching certainty (one chance in 163 that it might ultimately be proved inactive). In contrast, with any individual traditional remedy, our starting point is that we doubt whether it will be active, but once it produces a significant result, our faith in it is boosted a stage. However, the odds that it is genuinely active are still only 2:1 on, so we could hardly say that we have near-complete conviction – 'probable belief' is about as far as we could go.

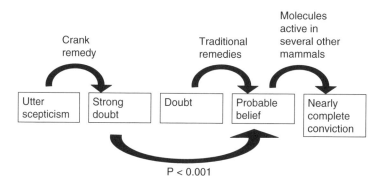

Figure 11.3   How a statistically significant result changes our beliefs about the existence of a treatment effect

This is where *P* values are perhaps of some value. A marginally significant result might take us one step up the ladder of belief, but if we get a result where the *P* value is extremely small (usually reported as *P* < 0.001), then that will provide a greater boost to our confidence – strong doubt might be converted into probable belief.

⚷ Significant results

A statistical result does not tell us what we should believe. It tells us how much we should change what we believe:

Non-significant – insufficient evidence to require any change.

Significant (*P* < 0.05) – increase credence to a useful extent.

Highly significant (*P* < 0.001) increase credence markedly.

11.2 Starting from extreme scepticism

Figure 11.3 suggests that, in the case of a crank remedy, where there is no rational expectation of therapeutic effectiveness, a significant outcome would still leave us in strong doubts as to its activity.

11.2.1 Comparing unlikeliness

It might seem unfair that we could obtain a significant result and yet still remain unconvinced that a treatment actually works. However, statistical significance only tells us that the results we obtained would be unlikely to arise if the null hypothesis were true. That does not automatically mean that we should start believing the alternative hypothesis. What we should do is to compare the relative likelihood of the two hypotheses.

If a quack medicine produced a greater effect than a placebo control and *P* = 0.01, then:

- it is hard to believe the null hypothesis, because the results we obtained would be unlikely to arise on that basis (one chance in 100 that such results would arise by sheer chance); however,

- it is also hard to believe the alternative hypothesis, because it posits activity where none would logically be expected (no exact figure is available, but there is probably far less than the one chance in a 100 seen above).

Neither theory is attractive, and all we can do is choose the one that is least unlikely; it is easier to believe that this was just a chance result and we still do not accept that the stuff works.

⊶⊙ Inherently unlikely treatments

If an experimental assessment of a highly improbable treatment produced a statistically significant result in favour of activity, the rational conclusion would be that you still do not believe it works.

11.2.2 Demonstrating the truth of apparently highly unlikely theories

It might appear that we are reverting to good old fashioned prejudice. If we already believe in something and we obtain a significant result, we continue to believe in it, but if we were sceptical to start with, we remain sceptical even after a significant result! However it is not that bad; we are just acknowledging that we are not starting from a blank sheet of paper. A significant result always moves us up one notch of credence. Even with the crank remedy, a significant result would leave us less sceptical and, if a series of well planned experiments continued to produce significant evidence of activity for this snake oil, then each of those trials would take our belief one notch up the scale. After three or four such trials, we would eventually have to accept that the wretched stuff does actually work.

11.3 Chapter summary

The interpretation of statistical significance must involve not only looking at the P value for the current experiment, but also taking stock of the previously available evidence as to whether two treatments are likely to give differing outcomes.

In a situation where there is already a strong empirical or rational basis for anticipating a difference, a significant result will leave us almost convinced that there is a real difference. Where there is less reason for anticipating an effect, a significant result will still increase our belief that there we are seeing a real difference, but some caution is still appropriate. In a situation where any difference in outcome is wildly unlikely, but we obtain statistically significant evidence in favour of an effect, we should remain sceptical and see whether a difference is confirmed in further experiments.

A model is proposed whereby statistically significant results always increase the credibility of a treatment effect, but precisely how convinced we become depends upon our prior assessment of the likelihood of a difference in outcomes.

12
The paired *t*-test – comparing two related sets of measurements

---

This chapter will . . .

- Describe the difference between paired and unpaired data

- Demonstrate that the paired *t*-test has greater power than the two-sample *t*-test when dealing with paired data

- Explain the source of its superior power

- Show how the paired *t*-test is performed

- Explore the merits of paired vs unpaired experimental designs

---

12.1 Paired data

There are many cases where we are faced with two columns of measured values and, as with previous examples, we want to see whether values are generally higher in one column than the other. Thus far, the situation is familiar. However, the data in the two columns may be related – they form natural pairs. In that case, the paired *t*-test provides a superior alternative to the two-sample *t*-test. An example follows:

Essential Statistics for the Pharmaceutical Sciences   Philip Rowe
© 2007 John Wiley & Sons, Ltd   ISBN 9780 470 03470 5 (HB)   ISBN 9780 470 03468 2 (PB)

12.1.1 Does a weight-loss drug really work?

An oral drug allegedly causes weight loss. We recruit 30 subjects who have received medical advice that they should loose weight. They all receive two periods of treatment each lasting 3 months. In one period patients receive placebo tablets and during the other they are given the active product. Each patient's weight is recorded at the end of both treatment periods. The results are shown in Table 12.1.

Table 12.1 Effects of an alleged weight reducing drug on subjects' weights

Subject number	Weight after placebo (kg)	Weight after active (kg)	Change in weight (active–placebo)(kg)
1	115.4	112.7	−2.7
2	118.9	113.8	−5.1
3	98.6	89.6	−9.0
4	108.3	93.1	−15.2
5	120.2	115.3	−4.9
6	115.0	112.3	−2.7
7	125.1	124.0	−1.1
8	120.4	115.6	−4.8
9	132.6	131.5	−1.1
10	100.8	98.9	−1.9
11	111.9	111.4	−0.5
12	105.3	103.0	−2.3
13	111.8	101.3	−10.5
14	98.0	91.3	−6.7
15	113.7	112.6	−1.1
16	117.1	118.2	+1.1
17	121.7	116.1	−5.6
18	123.6	127.5	+3.9
19	130.0	120.2	−9.8
20	128.0	117.3	−10.7
21	109.3	116.4	+7.1
22	117.7	113.8	−3.9
23	105.2	104.9	−0.3
24	120.3	123.4	+3.1
25	125.5	119.6	−5.9
26	114.3	106.4	−7.9
27	124.0	122.2	−1.8
28	123.3	123.8	+0.5
29	112.7	111.2	−1.5
30	113.8	106.6	−7.2
Mean	116.08	112.47	−3.62
SD	8.94	10.43	4.78

12.2 We could analyse the data using a two-sample *t*-test

We could analyse this data using the two-sample *t*-test. Comparing the weights at the end of the two treatment periods, we would obtain the following result:

Point estimate for difference in weight = −3.62 kg

95 per cent CI for difference = −8.64 to + 1.41 kg

The confidence interval includes zero, so the result is non-significant. The *P* value (0.155) confirms non-significance.

12.3 Using a paired *t*-test instead

12.3.1 Data variability

Table 12.1 also shows, for each subject, the difference between their two weighings. This has been calculated as weight after taking the active drug minus that after the placebo. In that way a negative figure indicates a weight loss.

Figure 12.1 shows (In the left panel) the weights at the end of both treatment periods. Each line connects an individual patient's post-placebo weight to that after active treatment. The vertical arrows emphasize the wide spread among these weights. However, the individual changes in weight (right panel) are markedly less spread out.

The difference in variability reflects the fact that some individuals may be much bigger than others, but those who start largest generally end largest and the smallest

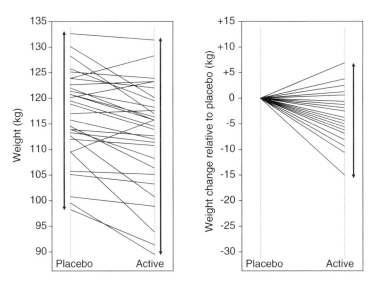

Figure 12.1 Greater variability among weights than among weight changes

end smallest. Consequently, the changes in weight do not show the extreme variation seen among the actual weights.

⚷ Changes less variable than the actual values

Where a series of individuals have widely differing values for an end-point, we may yet find that a treatment induces a relatively constant change in all individuals. In such a case, the actual values will have large SDs but the SD for the changes will be much smaller.

12.3.2   Reducing the variability we have to contend with

We know from Chapter 6 that data variability is a spoiler for *t*-tests and the large SDs for the weights in the first two columns of Table 12.1 are a prime contributor to the non-significant outcome of the two-sample *t*-test. It would be attractive to be able to base a statistical test solely on the column of weight changes, as these are considerably less variable. This is exactly what the paired *t*-test does.

12.4   Performing a paired *t*-test

12.4.1   Null and alternative hypotheses for the paired *t*-test

The calculation of a paired *t*-test is based on the changes in weight. The actual weights are, of course, necessary in order to calculate the changes, but once this has been done, only the changes are used.

The null hypothesis for the paired *t*-test will claim that, for a large group of subjects ('the population'), the mean weight change would be zero. It accepts that some individuals gain and others lose weight on the drug treatment, but it assumes that, in a large enough group, the gains and losses would cancel out. This implies that any apparent effect seen in our sample must be due to random sampling error.

The alternative hypothesis is that the drug does have an effect and that, however large a group we looked at, we would continue to see the effect.

⚷ Null and alternative hypotheses for a paired *t*-test

Null – the mean weight change in a large population of subjects would be zero.

Alternative - the mean weight change in a large population of subjects would *not* be zero.

Table 12.2 Generic output from paired *t*-test comparing weights after active and placebo drug treatment

Paired *t*-test:

	n	Mean
Active	30	112.47
Placebo	30	116.08
Differences	30	−3.62

95% CI for mean difference	−1.83 to −5.40
P	0.000

12.4.2 Calculation

To perform a paired *t*-test we simply calculate a 95 per cent CI for the mean among the weight changes (using final column of Table 12.1) and check to see whether the interval includes the value posited by the null hypothesis (zero).

Most statistical packages include this test. The two sets of data are usually entered into separate columns, with paired valued lying side-by-side. You then indicate the two relevant columns. With most implementations, you will not need to calculate the individual changes – this should be carried out as part of the procedure. Generic output is shown in Table 12.2, and this is illustrated in Figure 12.2.

A zero mean change, as claimed by the null hypothesis, is clearly excluded, so the result is statistically significant. The P value (<0.001) confirms the significance.

🔑 **Paired *t*-test is just a special use of a 95 per cent CI for a single set of values**

To perform a paired *t*-test we simply calculate a 95 per cent CI for mean individual change and check whether the interval includes zero.

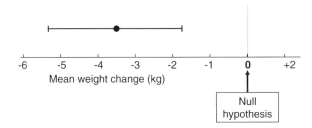

Figure 12.2 The 95 per cent confidence interval for the mean effect of the weight-loss drug

12.4.3   Different order of calculation in a paired *t*-test

In the two-sample *t*-test the two steps were:

1. calculation of the mean for each sample;

2. calculation of the 95 per cent CI for the difference between the two means.

For the paired *t*-test the order is reversed.

1. calculation of the change that has occurred within each pair of results;

2. calculation the 95 CI for the mean of these changes.

⇐◉ Order of calculation

Two-sample *t*-test – means, then difference of the means
Paired *t*-test – differences, then mean of the differences

12.5   What determines whether a paired *t*-test will be significant?

If you look at Figure 12.2, the outcome of the test will depend on two things:

- *How far from zero is the mean among the individual changes?* If the individual changes in weight are only small (or there is an approximate balance of positive and negative changes), the interval will be close to (and probably overlap) zero, making significance unlikely. With large changes in a consistent direction, the interval will be displaced well away from zero and the result should be significant.

- *How wide is the interval?* Small samples and/or high variability among the individual weight changes will make for a wide interval that is likely to cross zero, robbing us of significance.

This is summarised in Figure 12.3. The logic is very similar to that for the two-sample *t*-test, with one crucial difference. For a two-sample *t*-test, the variability that has to be considered is that among the two sets of weighings (the first two columns of data in Table 12.1). With a paired *t*-test, what matters is the variability among the individual weight changes (final column of Table 12.1). Therefore, with a paired *t*-test, the initial

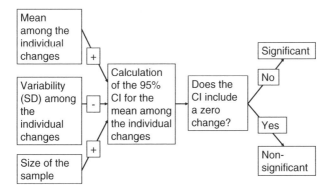

Figure 12.3   Factors influencing the outcome of a paired *t*-test

observations might be hideously variable, but if all individuals show similar changes, we can still obtain statistical significance.

12.6 Greater power of the paired *t*-test

When we initially applied a two-sample *t*-test to the first two columns of data in Table 12.1 (Section 12.2), the result was non-significant ($P = 0.155$), but the result of the paired *t*-test was clearly significant ($P < 0.001$). This is a typical example of the greater power of the paired *t*-test.

   Where data form natural pairs (as in the current example), it is very frequently the case that individuals who have the highest values under the first set of experimental conditions also have the highest values under the alternative conditions. As a result, the variability in the two original sets of data is greater than that among the individual changes that occur. This is the reason why the paired *t*-test is more powerful (often much more powerful) than the two-sample test.

12.7 The paired *t*-test is only applicable to naturally paired data

The whole logic of the paired *t*-test that we just performed was founded on the fact that we could calculate a change for each individual participant in the experiment and then use those changes to calculate the rest of the test. With the theophylline/ rifampicin experiment (Table 6.1), the data also consisted of two columns of data, but in that case there was no pairing. The first figure in the first column and that in the second column were derived from different individuals and it would have made no sense to start calculating the difference between these two figures and then move down to the second number in each column and so on.

   It is perhaps worth noting that the enhanced power of the paired *t*-test is dependent upon the data being genuinely paired. The paired test has no superiority where data lack natural pairing. So, if you have a set of data that are not genuinely paired and your two-sample *t*-test is non-significant, do not bother trying to concoct some artificial basis for claiming that the data are paired, just to allow a switch to the paired test. That particular manoeuvre is not only unjustified, but also ineffectual (it deserves a pirate box with zero pirate flags).

⚷ Greater power of the paired *t*-test

Where data is genuinely paired, the paired *t*-test is likely to be considerably more powerful than the two-sample test and should be employed.

If data is not naturally paired, the use of paired test is unjustified (and entirely pointless).

12.8 Choice of experimental design

Many experiments could be carried out either as paired or unpaired studies. For example the rifampicin/theophylline experiment (Table 6.1) was performed on an unpaired basis – 15 people received one treatment and a separate group of 15 received the other. This is referred to as a 'parallel groups' trial. We could have used a paired structure, with 15 subjects receiving one treatment on one occasion and the other treatment at some other time (a 'cross over' trial). The paired alternative would almost certainly have been a lot more powerful. However, it does not follow automatically that we should always be looking for a paired experimental design. The following points need to be born in mind:

12.8.1 In favour of paired designs – greater power

The use of a paired design produces data that can be analysed by the more powerful paired *t*-test, whereas data from an unpaired experiment can only be analysed by the less powerful two-sample *t*-test.

12.8.2 Against paired designs

Greater practical difficulties   In a paired design, each subject has to be studied twice. This may be slower to implement, especially if you need to leave a significant period of time between the two stages of the study. With human studies, there is also the problem that people may be less likely to volunteer if they know they will be experimented upon twice instead of just once.

Greater problems in the case of data loss If we used an unpaired design, we might find ourselves unable to obtain a measurement from one of our subjects. In that case, we would be left with 15 observations in one column, and only 14 in the other. With a two-sample *t*-test, we would still be able to use all of the data obtained. However, if we were performing a paired study (and presumably a paired *t*-test), we would not only lose that data point, but additionally its accompanying paired value would become useless and would have to be discarded.

The paired design may be logically impossible Some tests are destructive. For example, if we want to know whether a candidate drug causes liver enlargement in mice, we would need to compare organ weights after placebo and drug treatment. However, as the only practical way to determine liver weight is to kill the mouse and remove its liver, a paired experiment is going to be tricky.

⚷ Greater complexity of paired experimental designs

Paired experimental designs (which can be analysed by the more powerful paired *t*-test) may be more problematical than simple unpaired designs.

12.9 Requirements for applying a paired *t*-test

12.9.1 The column of individual changes should be consistent with a normal distribution

The paired *t*-test is just a special application of the 95 per cent CI for the mean and the requirement for normally distributed data, described in Chapter 5, applies in this case too. Just be aware that the confidence interval is calculated using the column of individual changes in weight (etc.), so it is these that need to be normally distributed. The subjects' placebo and active treated weights could be skewed or bimodal or any other horrible distribution – that would not matter. We just need the changes to be normal. As previously, we do not expect small samples to form perfect classic normal distributions, but if the column of individual changes shows extreme signs of non-normality, we should not trust a paired *t*-test (see Chapter 18 for possible solutions).

⚷ Requirement for performing a paired *t*-test

The individual changes must be consistent with a normal distribution. There is no need for the original observations to be normally distributed.

12.10 Sample sizes, practical significance and one-sided tests

Chapters 8–10 explained sample size calculations, practical significance and one-sided tests in detail and the point was made that these were general concepts that could be applied to a wide variety of tests. This section briefly reviews their application to the paired *t*-test.

12.10.1 Sample size calculations

The factors that influence necessary sample size for a paired *t*-test are very similar to those encountered with the two-sample test, but notice that we take into account variability among the individual changes in the end-point, not the two sets of initial observations. Below are reasonable values for the three relevant factors for our experiment on the effect of the weight-loss drug.

- *Size of effect to be detectable* – assume any weight change of less than 2 kg is of no medical or aesthetic relevance, so set the detection limit to this figure.

- *Variability in data* – we know that the sort of subject at whom the treatment is aimed will be constantly adopting and abandoning all manner of diets, so apart from anticipated variability among responses to the drug, there is also likely to be a lot of apparently random background noise. We allow for an SD among weight changes of ±4 kg.

- *Power* – a 90 per cent power is considered adequate.

If we feed these values into any statistical package that includes sample size calculations (e.g. Minitab), we will be told that a sample of 44 is required. However, remember that this is the amount of data we want to end up with and furthermore that paired designs can waste a lot of data if there are drop-outs, so realistically we need to start with 50 (or so) participants. This is another case where we were lucky to get away with what was in fact an underpowered experiment. Although numbers were inadequate, fortunately the drug caused a weight loss (3.62 kg) considerably greater than the minimum we wanted to be able to detect (2 kg).

12.10.2 Practically significant change, equivalence and non-inferiority testing

In Chapter 9, we saw the use of the two-sample *t*-test to answer questions such as 'Is the change big enough to matter?' or 'Can we demonstrate that there is no change of any consequence?' or 'Is this new product/procedure at least as good as the old one?' The paired *t*-test generates a 95 per cent CI for the treatment effect that can be combined with appropriate equivalence limits to answer precisely the same kinds of questions. The results are interpreted exactly as previously.

12.10.3 One tailed testing

As with the two-sample *t*-test, there may be circumstances where the question we want to answer concerns possible changes in some pre-determined direction. For example, with our weight-change experiment, the question posed might very reasonably have been 'Does the drug lead to a *loss* of weight?', since that would presumably be the motivation for using the drug. That question would be one-sided. As usual, the test could be converted to one-sidedness either by calculating a 90 per cent confidence interval and ignoring one limit or (if your statistical package allows) selecting a one-sided option. The usual rules apply – one-sided testing is fair enough so long as the decision to do so was made before the data were seen.

12.11 Summarizing the differences between the paired and two-sample *t*-tests

Table 12.3 summarizes the features that distinguish the paired from the two-sample *t*-test.

Table 12.3 Distinctions between the paired and the two-sample *t*-test

	Paired *t*-test	Two-sample *t*-test
Methodology	1. Calculate the difference for each pair of values	1. Calculate the mean for each column
	2. Calculate CI for the mean of these differences	2. Calculate CI for the difference between these two means
Use with unpaired data?	Unjustified and pointless	Correct procedure
Use with paired data?	Correct procedure	Possible, but a poor choice – lacks power
Use if unequal numbers of observations in the two columns?	Impossible – data evidently not paired!	No problem, except slight loss of power

12.12 Chapter summary

The paired *t*-test is used where data form natural pairs. Its classic use arises when we have observed the same individual (human or otherwise) under two different circumstances (before vs after treatment or placebo treatment period vs active treatment period, etc).

For each individual we calculate the difference in the measured value, under the two circumstances. These individual changes are then used to calculate a 95 per cent CI for the mean effect. If the interval excludes zero, the result is statistically significant.

The paired *t*-test offers the greatest advantage over the two-sample *t*-test when values are much higher in some individuals than in others, but all individuals show roughly the same change. In such cases, the two-sample test would be degraded by the extreme variation between individuals, but the paired test would only have to cope with the lesser variation among the individual changes.

It is always worth considering the use of a paired experimental design, as it will allow the use of the more powerful paired *t*-test. However, paired experiments can present practical difficulties that may outweigh this statistical advantage. For a valid paired *t*-test, the individual changes in the measured parameter should form a normal distribution.

General statistical methods such as sample size estimation, determination of practical significance and one-sided testing can be applied to the paired *t*-test in the same manner that we have already seen for the two-sample *t*-test.

13

Analyses of variance – going beyond *t*-tests

This chapter will . . .

- Describe how experimental design is described in terms of 'factors' and 'levels'

- Show the use of the one-way analysis of variance to analyse experiments where there is only one experimental factor, but it takes three or more levels

- Describe the use of 'follow up tests' to discover which treatments differ from which others

- Describe the two-way analysis of variance where two experimental factors have been investigated in parallel

- Explain the concept of 'interaction' between factors

- Show that experiments should not include unnecessary levels as these can dilute the contrast between other treatments that do differ, causing a loss of statistical significance

Essential Statistics for the Pharmaceutical Sciences   Philip Rowe
© 2007 John Wiley & Sons, Ltd   ISBN 9780 470 03470 5 (HB)   ISBN 9780 470 03468 2 (PB)

13.1 Extending the complexity of experimental designs

With *t*-tests, we can compare two sets of data. There are other experimental designs which will require a comparison of more than two sets of data and that is when we need an 'analysis of variance' (AoV or ANOVA). Traditional statistics books always get their knickers in a frightful twist trying to explain ANOVAs. It is difficult to imagine why, because they are actually quite minor extensions of the two-sample *t*-test.

13.1.1 Factors and levels

A 'factor' is something that we manipulate as part of an experiment in order to see whether it alters the endpoint we are measuring. In the rifampicin/theophylline experiment (Chapter 6), the factor was rifampicin. We then say that the factor has a number of 'levels'. This is the number of different possibilities for that factor. There were two levels for rifampicin – it was either administered or withheld. In the weight-loss experiment in the previous chapter, there was again just one factor (drug) and it also had two levels (used or not used). In fact, for any experiment that can be analysed by a *t*-test there is always one experimental factor for which there are just two levels – the simplest of all experimental designs.

⌐◎ 'Factors', 'levels' and analyses of variance

A 'factor' is an aspect of our experimental design that will be deliberately altered to see how this affects the outcome. Each different possibility within a factor is a 'level'.

    t-Tests are used for the simplest possible experimental designs, i.e. a single factor with just two levels. Analyses of variance are used for any design of greater complexity.

13.2 One-way analysis of variance

13.2.1 A single experimental factor

In our first step up the ladder of complexity we will stick with just one experimental factor, but consider cases where that factor has more than two levels.

    As an example, we want to improve the chemical synthesis of a drug. It is already known that finely divided platinum is a good catalyst for the reaction, but we want to investigate the potential use of other related metals. We therefore perform the synthesis of the drug under fixed conditions of pressure, temperature, etc., but vary the catalyst added. The metals investigated are platinum, palladium, iridium and rhodium and additionally an alloy of palladium and iridium. Five replicate

Table 13.1 Effect of catalyst on yield (percentage of theoretical maximum)

	Platinum	Palladium	Iridium	Palladium–Iridium	Rhodium
	11.3	15.4	12.1	13.1	12.0
	10.7	17.0	12.2	13.7	11.6
	9.8	18.4	13.1	13.5	9.1
	10.4	17.5	11.8	14.0	11.9
	11.5	18.8	10.4	14.2	11.3
Mean	10.74	17.42	11.92	13.70	11.18
SD	0.69	1.34	0.98	0.43	1.20

syntheses are carried out using each catalyst. The yields obtained (expressed as percentages of the theoretically achievable yield) are shown in Table 13.1.

13.2.2 Do not perform multiple *t*-tests

A seductively simple way to analyse the data would be to say that platinum is our current standard catalyst, so it makes sense to treat platinum as a control and compare it against each alternative in turn, using a series of two-sample *t*-tests. However, this would involve performing four separate tests. We know that, for every statistical test performed, there is a 5 per cent risk of a false positive. With a simple experiment like the weight loss study (Chapter 12), only one test is performed and the chance of a false positive is an acceptable 5 per cent. However, in this case we would be performing four tests each carrying a 5 per cent risk and the chances of hitting a false positive at some stage would be a lot more than 5 per cent. (The risk is not quite as bad as the simplistic 4×5 per cent $= 20$ per cent, but it is well in excess of 15 per cent.) The general term for such repeated analyses with their attendant risk of false positives is 'multiple testing', and it is a problem that can raise its ugly head in a wide range of statistical scenarios. (Chapter 18 considers other forms of multiple testing.)

 Multiple testing

When results from several treatments are to be compared, multiple *t*-tests should not be used – this leads to increased risk of false positives.

Instead we need a single test that will consider the whole data set and deliver a single verdict. The appropriate test is called the 'one-way analysis of variance'. The 'one-way' part of the name reflects the fact that there is still only one factor under investigation (in this case, which catalyst to use).

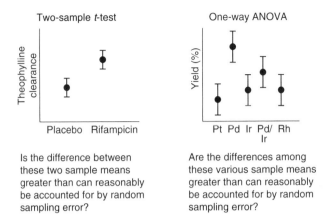

Figure 13.1   The one-way analysis of variance as a minor extension of the two-sample *t*-test

---

🔑 One-way analysis of variance

Is used when:

• the end point is a measured value (generally on an interval scale);

• there is one experimental factor;

• the factor has three or more levels.

Figure 13.1 shows that the application of a one-way ANOVA to this data is only a minor extension of what we already did with the rifampicin/theophylline clearances and a two-sample *t*-test.

13.2.3   Null and alternative hypotheses

The null hypothesis must deny that any of the catalysts differs from any of the others.

🔑 Null and alternative hypotheses

Null – in the long term, the mean yield of product would be the same for all five
   catalysts.
Alternative – in the long term, at least one of the catalysts would produce a different
   mean yield from one of the others.

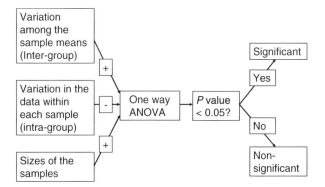

Figure 13.2   Factors influencing the outcome of a one-way ANOVA

The mechanism implied by the null hypothesis is also just an extension of that discussed in relation to the *t*-test. It is assumed that the five catalysts are in reality indistinguishable, but within these small samples, random sampling error has led to an illusion of variability in their effectiveness. Presumably, the effectiveness of some catalysts has been overestimated and/or that of others understated.

13.2.4   What governs whether a significant result will emerge?

Since the function of the one-way ANOVA is so similar to the of the two-sample *t*-test, it is no great surprise that the factors that govern its outcome are also virtually identical. They are shown in Figure 13.2. In considering this diagram, we need to keep a close eye on the term 'variation'. There are two types.

Intra-group variation   The five individual results listed under 'platinum' in Table 13.1 were all gathered under conditions that were intended to be, as far as possible, identical. However, each time we repeat the experiment, some variation always creeps in. Variation within a group of replicates is called 'intra-group variation'.

Inter-group variation   There are also overall differences between groups as reflected by the mean yields for each type of catalyst. This is termed 'inter-group variation'. There will always be a degree of inter-group variation, even if all the catalysts are exactly equally effective, because of random sampling error. However, if there are real differences in the effectiveness of the various catalysts, inter-group variation will be boosted beyond the level we would expect to arise from random sampling error alone.

Plus and minus signs in Figure 13.2   The plus and minus signs in Figure 13.2 reflect the effect of each aspect on the likelihood of a significant outcome and are assigned as follows:

- *Differences between the sample means (inter-group variation)* – small differences may only reflect random sampling error, but if the sample means differ widely, a significant conclusion is more likely.

- *Variability in the data within samples (intra-group variation)* – if the data within each sample are highly variable, random error will be increased and we will be less convinced that any apparent differences between catalysts are real.

- *Sample sizes* – large samples should produce less random error and we will be more confident that any inter-group variation is due to real differences among the catalysts.

13.2.5   Performing a one way analysis of variance

With most statistics packages, data that are to be subjected to a one-way analysis of variance are entered into two columns in a similar way to that seen with a two-sample *t*-test (Section 6.8). One column contains a series of codes indicating what catalyst was used and the other column contains the corresponding experimental results. In the first five rows, the results are labelled as being due to the use of platinum (Pt), the next five are due to palladium (Pd) and so on. The general appearance will be as in Table 13.2.

To carry out the test, you will need to indicate which column contains the codes and which the actual data. The output varies considerably between packages, but almost all will provide that shown in Table 13.3 as a minimum.

Table 13.2   Generalized method for entering data into statistics packages in preparation for a one-way analysis of variance

Column 1 Catalyst	Column 2 Yield
Pt	11.3
Pt	10.7
Pt	9.8
Pt	10.4
Pt	11.5
Pd	15.4
Pd	17.0
Pd	18.4
Pd	17.5
Pd	18.8
Ir	12.1
Ir	12.2
etc.	etc.

Table 13.3 Generic output for one-way analysis of variance of effect of catalyst on reaction efficiency

One-way analysis of variance

End-point: Yield
Factor: Catal

Source	DF	SS	MS	*F*	*P*
Catalyst	4	148.062	37.016	38.37	0.000
Error	20	19.296	0.965		
Total	24	67.358			

The reporting of analyses of variance is traditionally an ugly business, including a mass of intermediate working that is of limited value in most circumstances. If we ignore all the dross, the *P* value is given as '0.000' (i.e. <0.001) which is statistically clearly significant.

13.2.6 Follow up tests – interpreting significance

A *P* value well below 0.05 means that we have strong evidence against the null hypothesis. However, even if we are happy to exclude the null hypothesis, Figure 13.3 shows that we are still left with a wide range of possible alternatives. It could be [part (b) of Figure 13.3] that just one catalyst is different and all the others are indistinguishable, or (c) they might break up into two groups, or (d) they might all be different from each other, and so on. We are left with several dozen possibilities. The

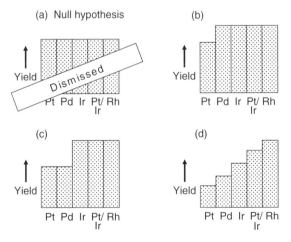

Figure 13.3 Interpreting a significant result from a one-way ANOVA

significant result from the ANOVA is rather frustrating – it tells us there are some differences in there somewhere, but it is not telling us where they lie.

The means and SDs for each catalyst (Table 13.1) suggest that the main features are palladium producing higher yields than any other metal, with palladium–iridium a good second and little to choose between the others. However, we really need a more objective assessment and this is where 'follow up' tests come in. They are called 'follow up' tests because traditionally they are only applied after an ANOVA has proved significant, although there is no strict need to follow that sequence. There are innumerable follow-up tests available, but the two outlined below will cope with most situations.

Dunnett's test   With Dunnett's test, we select one of the treatments as a 'control' or 'reference' group. All other groups are then compared against the control. In our case we might declare platinum to be the control and then compare all other treatments against it – a total of four comparisons.

Tukey's test   Here, all groups are compared with all other groups in every possible pairing. With our data set, we would have to compare the first treatment against four others, the next against three others, and so on, giving a total of $4 + 3 + 2 + 1 = 10$ comparisons.

Performing Tukey's test   With our experiment, a case could be made for performing either a Dunnett's or a Tukey's test. The general rule, that choices of statistical methodology should be made in advance of seeing the data, includes the selection of a follow-up test. Let us assume that a decision had been made that we would use Tukey's test.

In most statistical packages, the implementation of the analysis of variance includes an option to select a Tukey's test. The format of the output varies enormously, but (as in Table 13.4) should include a list of confidence intervals for the difference between each possible pair of catalysts. Each line of output shows the difference calculated as the yield with the first metal minus that with the second. The results are shown ordered according to yield [palladium (highest) to platinum (lowest)].

The output begins with palladium and it is contrasted with all four other catalysts. In each case the figures are positive (palladium is superior) and the CI for the difference excludes zero, so all comparisons are statistically significant. Palladium is demonstrably superior to all the competition, even its nearest rival – palladium–iridium.

Next, there is a block comparing palladium–iridium with all other catalysts except palladium (already considered). In this case, the gap between palladium–iridium and it is nearest rival (iridium) is just a little too small to be statistically significant; however, the alloy was shown to be superior to the other two metals. For all the remaining comparisons among iridium, rhodium and platinum, the interval includes zero and they are non-significant.

Table 13.4 Generic output from Tukey's test, showing confidence limits for the differences between pairs of catalysts (percentage points)

Tukey's test

Confidence Intervals: 99.28%

	Lower limit for difference	Upper limit for difference	Significant?
Palladium–palladium/iridium	+1.86	+5.58	Significant
Palladium–iridium	+3.64	+7.36	Significant
Palladium–rhodium	+4.38	+8.10	Significant
Palladium–platinum	+4.82	+8.54	Significant
Palladium/iridium–iridium	−0.08	+3.64	Non-significant
Palladium/iridium–rhodium	+0.66	+4.38	Non-significant
Palladium/iridium–platinum	+1.10	+4.82	Significant
Iridium–rhodium	−1.12	+2.60	Non-significant
Iridium–platinum	−0.68	+3.04	Non-significant
Rhodium–platinum	−1.42	+2.30	Non-significant

Initially, this seems to be a confusing jumble of information, but Figure 13.4 should make sense of it. The metals are ordered according to their effectiveness (this time going from least to most effective). For the first three metals (Pt, Rh and Ir), all comparisons among them were non-significant, so a horizontal bar indicates that these three metals are not statistically distinguishable. Another bar shows our failure to demonstrate a significant difference between iridium and the alloy, but notice that neither of these bars covers all four metals, because the contrast between platinum and rhodium at one extreme and the palladium–iridium alloy at the other was great enough to be significant. Palladium is not covered by any bars, as it is distinguishable from all other metals.

Practical significance
The ANOVA only tested statistical significance. However, Tukey's test reports confidence intervals for the sizes of the various differences, so we can also assess whether any increase in yield that might be achieved by a change of catalyst would be big enough to be of practical significance.

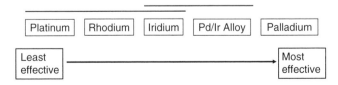

Figure 13.4 Groups of catalysts that are not statistically distinguishable

---

━○ Dunnett's and Tukey's follow-up tests

The analysis of variance only tells us whether there are any differences among the available treatments. It does not tell us either:

• which treatment differs from which other; or

• the extent of the difference between any pair of treatments.

Follow-up tests rectify both of these shortcomings.
Dunnett's – compares one control group against all others.
Tukey's – compares all groups against all others.

Have we not just resorted to multiple testing?   Earlier (Section 13.2.2) we rehearsed arguments suggesting that it would be wrong to carry out multiple *t*-tests, as this would increase the risk of false positives. Does not the same objection apply to Tukey's test, since it incorporates 10 individual comparisons? The answer is no. Tukey's test is designed to produce a 'test-wide error rate' of 5 per cent. What this means is that there is a total risk of 5 per cent that we might produce one (or more) false positive findings. This is achieved, by having each individual comparison performed to a higher standard of proof, guaranteeing that any one comparison will carry much less than a 5 per cent risk. By the time we have performed all 10 comparisons, we will have accumulated a total risk of 5 per cent. In many statistical packages, the output for Tukey's test includes a statement of the level of confidence for each individual comparison. With our catalyst experiment, 99.28 per cent confidence intervals are used. The chances of a false positive arising from any given contrast is therefore $100 - 99.28 = 0.72$ per cent. By the time we have performed all 10 comparisons, the total risk accumulates to the standard (and acceptable) 5 per cent.

Performing Dunnett's test   In the real world, it would be naughty to start doing a Dunnett's test at this stage, since we have already seen the data and had previously committed ourselves to Tukey's test. However, just so you can see the procedure, we will perform Dunnett's test with platinum as control.

If you select the option for Dunnett's test in your statistical package, you will additionally have to indicate that platinum is to act as the control. The generic output (Table 13.5) shows the difference of each metal in turn from platinum. Platinum is demonstrated to be inferior to palladium and the alloy, but there is no statistically significant evidence of a difference from rhodium or iridium.

If your package indicates the level of confidence used, it should be 98.47 per cent. This means that the individual error rate for each comparison is 1.53 per cent. This is higher than the corresponding figure (0.72 per cent) for Tukey's test. The reason for this is that we are now performing only four comparisons instead of 10 and so individual comparisons do not need to be performed to quite such high standards.

Table 13.5 Generic output from Dunnett's test, showing confidence limits for the differences between platinum and the other catalysts (percentage points)

Dunnett's test

Control: platinum

Confidence Intervals: 98.47%

	Lower limit for difference	Upper limit for difference	Significant?
Rhodium–platinum	−1.21	+2.09	Non-significant
Iridium–platinum	−0.47	+2.83	Non-significant
Palladium/iridium–platinum	+1.31	+4.61	Significant
Palladium–platinum	+5.03	+8.33	Significant

When planning experiments, it is worth remembering that, as the number of treatments increases, there is a very steep increase in the number of comparisons that Tukey's test would make and the individual comparisons will have to be carried out to correspondingly high standards of proof.

⚷ Test-wide error rate remains at 5 per cent

When Tukey's or Dunnett's test make multiple comparisons, each of these is performed to a higher than normal standard of proof, so that the accumulative risk of generating any false positives remains at the usual 5 per cent.

13.2.7 Balanced data

The data from our catalyst experiment are 'balanced', i.e. there are exactly equal numbers of replicates for each catalyst. This is not a requirement for the one-way ANOVA and, if a small amount of data loss occurs, the analysis can still go ahead. For any given number of observations, the power of the ANOVA will be greatest with a balanced data set and this is also true for Tukey's test. The only circumstance where power will be greater with an imbalanced data set is where a Dunnett's test is planned. Here, the control group is of special importance because it is used in all the comparisons. For this test, it is worthwhile trying to generate some extra data for the control group.

13.2.8 Requirements for performing analyses of variance

The requirements are similar to those for the two-sample t-test. Each set of data should be drawn from a normally distributed population and they should all have the same SD. Small samples never exactly fit these requirements, but gross deviations from the ideal can cause real difficulties. In severe cases, the data needs to be transformed to normality (Section 5.10) or an alternative method such as the Kruskal–Wallis test can be substituted for the one-way ANOVA (Chapter 17).

13.3 Two-way analysis of variance

13.3.1 Investigating two experimental factors simultaneously

The final step up the ladder of complexity is the simultaneous consideration of more than one experimental factor. With our drug synthesis experiment, where we considered different catalysts, we might also want to vary the method of mixing during the reaction. In the experiment presented in Table 13.1, mixing was achieved by stirring, but we suspect that this may be inadequate and that ultrasonication might break up aggregated material more effectively. Table 13.6 shows the factors and levels that we will consider.

Our experiment will then investigate all possible combinations of these two factors, i.e. $5 \times 2 = 10$ combinations. When we use all combinations of two (or more) factors, it is called a 'full factorial experiment'. We used five replicates of each combination and the results are shown in Table 13.7.

The appropriate statistical test for two experimental factors and a full factorial design is the two-way analysis of variance.

⚙️ Two way analysis of variance

Is used when:

- The end point is a measured value (generally on an interval scale).

- There are two experimental factors.

- All possible combinations of the two factors have been studied (full factorial experiment).

Table 13.6 Factors and levels to be considered

Factor	Levels
Catalyst – five levels	Pt, Pd, Ir, Pd/Ir, Rh
Mixing – two levels	Stirring, ultrasonication

Table 13.7 Effects of catalyst and mixing method on yield (percentage of theoretical maximum)

	Platinum	Palladium	Iridium	Palladium–iridium	Rhodium
	11.1	15.9	10.9	14.1	13.0
	11.7	18.9	13.4	13.9	12.3
Stirred	9.8	18.9	10.5	14.2	11.0
	12.1	15.5	12.2	13.5	9.9
	9.3	17.2	10.9	14.0	10.6
	12.8	20.0	14.8	16.3	13.1
	13.8	19.9	11.9	17.2	13.4
Ultrasonic	12.3	19.5	15.3	16.0	13.8
	12.4	20.5	14.3	15.1	13.6
	12.0	18.3	15.2	17.0	12.8

13.3.2 Interaction

When we analyse the data, we will obviously be looking to see whether altering the catalyst or altering the mixing method changes the yield. However, with more than one factor, we will also need to check for something new – interaction. This is most easily explained by looking at the results of our experiment. We start by calculating the mean result for each set of five replicates and these are shown in Table 13.8. These can then be presented graphically – see Figure 13.5.

Changing the mixing method does seem to have an effect on the yield – for each metal, the yield is always higher with ultrasonication than with stirring and, further-more, the increase in yield when we switch to ultrasonication is fairly consistent for all five metals – an increase of around 2–3 per cent. Because the increase in yield is about the same for all five metals, we say that there the effects of the catalyst and stirring are simply 'additive' and there is no interaction between the two factors. If ultrasonica-tion caused a much greater increase in yield with some metals than with others, interaction would be present.

> ## ⚷ Interaction
>
> Interaction is present when the effect produced by changing the level of one factor is dependent upon the level of another factor.

Table 13.8 Mean yield for each combination of catalyst and stirring method (%)

	Pt	Pd	Ir	Pd–Ir	Rh
Stirred	10.80	17.28	11.58	13.94	11.36
Ultrasonic	12.66	19.64	14.30	16.32	13.34

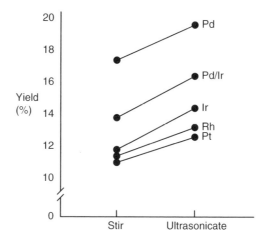

Figure 13.5   Effect of catalyst and mixing method on yield

Graphical check for interaction   We can make a visual check for interaction by looking for parallel lines in a graph like Figure 13.5. Two possible outcomes are shown in Figure 13.6. In the left-hand graph, the boost in yield that results from the use of ultrasonication is exactly the same for all metals (parallel lines – no interaction), but on the right-hand side, there is only a tiny change with platinum compared with that seen with the palladium–iridium alloy (non-parallel lines – interaction).

The points plotted in Figure 13.5 are of course only sample means and they are subject to the usual random sampling error. We cannot arrive at any definitive conclusions just by looking at such a graph. If the points for ultrasonication were only slightly higher than those for stirring, the difference could be nothing more than sampling error. Similarly, slight non-parallelism may not be real interaction, but just

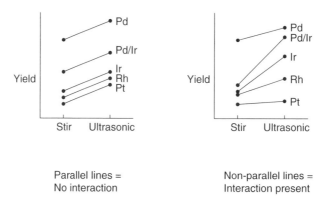

Figure 13.6   Visual check for interaction

more sampling error. We need a two-way analysis of variance to see whether such features within the data are sufficiently clear cut to convince us they are real.

13.3.3 Null hypotheses

In this case, we will be testing three null hypotheses:

- The long-term mean yield would be the same with all five catalysts.

- The long-term mean yield would be the same with both mixing methods.

- There is no interaction between the two factors.

These are independent hypotheses. We could end up accepting them all, rejecting them all or accepting some and rejecting others.

13.3.4 Performing a two-way ANOVA

We enter the data into a stats package in a similar way to that seen in Table 13.2, except that we now need an additional column to contain codes for the mixing method (the additional column can be seen in Table 13.9).

Table 13.9 Generalized method for entering data into statistics packages in preparation for a two-way analysis of variance

Column 1 Catal	Column 2 Mixing	Column 3 Yield
Pt	Stir	11.1
Pt	Stir	11.7
Pt	Stir	9.8
Pt	Stir	12.1
Pt	Stir	9.3
Pd	Stir	15.9
Pd	Stir	18.9
.	.	.
.	.	.
Pt	Ultra	12.8
Pt	Ultra	13.8
Pt	Ultra	12.3
Pt	Ultra	12.4
Pt	Ultra	12.0
Pd	Ultra	20.0
Pd	Ultra	19.9
etc.	etc.	etc.

Table 13.10 Generic output for two-way analysis of variance of effect of catalyst and mixing method on reaction efficiency

Two-way analysis of variance
End-point
End-point: yield
Fixed factors(s): Catal, Mixing
Random factor(s):

Source	DF	SS	MS	F	P
Catal	4	300.931	75.2327	67.41	0.000
Mixing	1	63.845	63.8450	57.20	0.000
Interaction	4	1.186	0.2965	0.27	0.898
Error	40	44.644	1.1161		
Total	49	410.606			

The detailed method for conducting a two-way analysis of variance varies from one stats package to another, but with all packages the output, should include all the usual ANOVA rubbish, along with the three P values that we really want (Table 13.10).

13.3.5   Interpretation of a two-way ANOVA in the absence of interaction

The three rows to look at are those beginning 'Catal', 'Mixing' and 'Interaction'. The first two give the results for the effects of changing the catalyst and for changing the mixing method. The third row reports on the possibility of interaction between these two factors. Catalyst and mixing method are confirmed as clearly significant ($P < 0.001$), but a P value of 0.898 provides no evidence of interaction and we can reasonably go ahead with some fairly sweeping and simple interpretations of the effects of both factors.

So far as mixing is concerned, we can say that ultrasonication is always superior to stirring, whatever catalyst is being used. Also, since there is no evidence of interaction, we can produce a single estimate of the extent of the improvement we achieve by using ultrasonication. From Table 13.8 we can calculate the gain with platinum as $12.66 - 10.80 = 1.86$ per cent and so on. See Table 13.11.

The extent of the superiority of ultrasonication over stirring is an increase in yield of about 2.3 per cent. The results for the catalysts essentially confirm what we already knew, with palladium being the most effective.

13.3.6   Balanced data

Like the single-factor experiment (Table 13.1), this experiment is also balanced – there were equal numbers of replicates for each combination of factors.

Table 13.11 Increases in yield due to the use of ultrasonication instead of stirring (%)

Metal	Increase in yield (%)
Pt	1.86
Pd	2.36
Ir	2.72
Pd–Ir	2.38
Rh	1.98
Mean	2.26%

The classic two-way ANOVA does demand a balanced data set. It can therefore be a pain if a piece of data is lost. However, there is a technique called a general linear model that will achieve the same ends as the two-way ANOVA, without the need for perfectly balanced data. Many statistical packages offer the technique.

⚷ Summary

- There is no significant evidence of interaction between the two factors ($P = 0.898$).

- There is significant evidence that yield varies according to the mixing method used ($P < 0.001$). Ultrasonication produces a yield around 2.3 per cent greater than that achieved by stirring.

- There is significant evidence confirming our previous conclusion that yield varies according to which catalyst is used ($P < 0.001$).

13.3.7 Two-way ANOVA with interaction

In the next example we investigated the effects of punch design and compression force on the tensile strength of tablets made from hydroxymethylpropylcellulose (HPMC). Tablets are produced using low or high compression force (10 or 20 kN) and three different designs for the metal punches that form the tablets. A full factorial design therefore required six combinations of the two factors. Each combination was studied using six replicates. The results are shown in Table 13.12 and Figure 13.7.

Figure 13.7 strongly suggests interaction, with the higher compression force always increasing tablet strength, but its advantage over the lower force is fairly marginal with punch type A, and much more marked with punch C. These results were analysed using a two-way ANOVA and the main results are shown in Table 13.13.

Table 13.12   Effects of punch design and compression force on tablet strength (MPa)

	Punch A		Punch B		Punch C	
Low force	4.00		6.49		7.92	
	4.79		8.35		8.15	
	5.50	Mean	6.40	Mean	7.60	Mean
	5.15	5.208	6.37	7.092	9.64	8.753
	5.26		6.86		9.98	
	6.55		8.08		9.23	
High force	4.90		9.63		14.60	
	4.90		9.67		13.81	
	5.04	Mean	8.72	Mean	13.20	Mean
	6.93	5.787	8.08	9.075	14.62	13.863
	7.13		10.25		13.77	
	5.82		8.10		13.18	

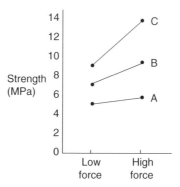

Figure 13.7   Effect of punch design and compression force on tablet strength – quantitative interaction

Table 13.13   Generic output for two-way analysis of variance of effect of punch designs and compression force on tablet strength

Two-way analysis of variance

End-point: strength
Fixed factors(s): Force, Punch
Random factor(s):

Source	DF	SS	MS	F	P
Force	1	58.854	58.854	74.21	0.000
Punch	2	203.412	101.706	128.23	0.000
Interaction	2	32.286	16.143	20.35	0.000
Error	30	23.794	0.793		
Total	35	318.346			

The statistical analysis confirms the presence of interaction ($P < 0.001$). We will therefore need to be more circumspect in our interpretation. We can still rank the various levels of the factors. Strength is always greatest with the use of the higher force and it always increases as we go from punch A to B and then C. What we can no longer do is to make any across-the-board assessment of the extent of these superiorities. For example, using high compression force increases strength by only about 0.5 MPa with punch A, but the increase is in excess of 5 MPa with punch C. This type of interaction, where the effect of changing from one treatment to another, always produces a change in one direction, but the extent of the change is variable is called 'quantitative interaction'.

🔑 Summary

- There is significant evidence of interaction between the two factors ($P < 0.001$).

- There is significant evidence that strength varies according to compression force ($P < 0.001$). High pressure always produces the greater strength.

- There is significant evidence that strength varies according to punch design ($P < 0.001$). Punch C produces the greatest strength and punch A the least.

- It is not possible to make any general statement about how much extra strength arises from the use of the higher compression force nor about the extent of the difference that arises from using (say) punch C instead of B.

- This is an example of quantitative interaction.

13.3.8 Quantitative vs qualitative interaction

In the tabletting example there was interaction and as a result we could no longer make any general statement about (for example) the extent of the increase in tablet strength brought about by changing the compression force. However, we were at least able to comment on the direction of change – greater force always caused greater strength to some degree. The real nightmare is the sort of hypothetical result suggested in Figure 13.8.

We now have two punch designs (B and C) where increased pressure leads to stronger tablets, but punch A responds in exactly the opposite manner. The (very) non-parallel lines again indicate interaction, but now in a much nastier form. With this sort of messy outcome, we cannot even produce any across-the-board comment on the direction of change that will arise from increased compression pressure, let alone the size of the change.

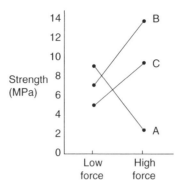

Figure 13.8 Qualitative interaction between punch design and compression force

If what we saw in Figure 13.7 was 'quantitative interaction', then Figure 13.8 may be said to show 'qualitative interaction'.

🔑 Interpreting results in the presence of interaction

Type of interaction	General statement of the *direction* of difference when changing from one treatment to another?	General statement of the *size* of difference when changing from one treatment to another?
None	Yes	Yes
Quantitative	Yes	No
Qualitative	No	No

13.3.9 Diagnosing the nature of interaction

If evidence of interaction is significant, a graph such as Figure 13.7 or 13.8 will illustrate the nature of the interaction (quantitative or qualitative). The *P* value will only tell you whether interaction is present, not what form it takes.

13.4 Multi-factorial experiments

There is no logical reason why we need to stop at two experimental factors. When trying to optimize a drug synthesis we might need to define the best:

- catalyst;

- mixing method;

- concentrations of reactants;

- temperature;

- pressure;

- reaction time.

A full factorial experiment could then involve hundreds of combinations and be completely unrealistic. Fortunately there are compromise designs called 'fractional factorial designs' that can be used so long as we are prepared to make reasonable assumptions that interactions will not be excessive. Statistical analyses are then available to tease out which factors really are significant and to determine what combination of levels produces the optimum outcome. The design and analysis of such experiments goes well beyond the scope of this book, but many statistical packages provides all the methodology for rational optimization (Minitab is especially good at this) – all you need is a competent statistician to hold your hand.

13.5 Keep it simple – keep it powerful

13.5.1 Significant results can be lost by dilution

Figure 13.9 shows a series of clinical trials for drugs designed to reduce blood pressure. The vertical axis shows the mean change in pressure caused by each

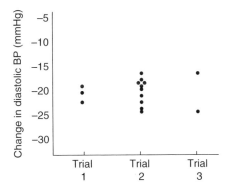

Figure 13.9 Changes in blood pressure when comparing three or 10 identical products (trials 1 and 2) or two genuinely differing products (trial 3)

product. Trial 1 compared just three products, whereas the second looked at 10. If there were no real difference among the products, but we suffered the usual random sampling error, we would expect to see clusters of similar, but slightly dispersed, points. Within each trial, there will always be one treatment that happens to produce the greatest and another the least response. With greater numbers of products being compared, there will be an increasing likelihood that abnormally large and small responses will arise by chance. So, the fact that there is a greater spread of treatment effects in trial 2 than in trial 1 does not necessarily provide any greater evidence of inter-product variability – we would expect a greater spread with more products.

Trial 3 used only two products and the difference in their effectiveness is the same as the maximum contrast in trial 2. However, this is now much more impressive evidence, because the chances that two products would generate such a difference are far less than would be the case among 10.

This means that there is a danger that two genuinely different treatments might fail to be detected as such if they are accompanied by a mass of other treatments. There might be a large difference in the results for the two products, but it would be dismissed as non-significant – merely a difference you would expect to find among a large number of products.

13.5.2 An example of dilution

We can illustrate the doleful effect of dilution without resorting to such extremes as experiments with 10 different products. Just increasing the number of treatments from two to three can wreck an experiment.

Our real intention is to investigate a possible difference in effectiveness of two formulations (A and B) of the same beta-blocker (a drug that reduces blood pressure). However, we are persuaded to include a third formulation (C), making a three-armed trial. Thirty-six patients are randomized into three groups and then all have a period taking a placebo and a period taking one of the formulations of the beta-blocker. For each patient, we calculate the reduction in diastolic pressure caused by taking the active drug. The reductions in blood pressure are shown in Table 13.14. When the data are submitted to a one-way analysis of variance, the *P* value is 0.067 and therefore non-significant.

The tragedy is that the original interest was in formulations A and B, which have emerged as quite strongly contrasting (see means in Table 13.14), but with the inclusion of the additional formulation C, they are now just the most contrasting among three and the difference is inadequate for statistical significance.

As a matter of interest, we could run a two-sample *t*-test on the formulations in which we were really interested. The resulting *P* value (0.025) is comfortably significant. Apart from sabotaging the brakes on the car of whoever persuaded you to include the extra formulation, there is nothing that can be done about the failure at this stage. We had committed to including all three formulations and using an

Table 13.14   Reductions in blood pressure (mmHg) when patients take a formulation (A, B or C) of a beta-blocker

	A	B	C
	21	23	31
	13	22	19
	24	29	23
	26	33	15
	16	21	26
	29	25	28
	28	20	18
	17	30	31
	18	30	30
	20	22	19
	29	35	20
	17	32	22
Mean	21.50	26.83	23.50

ANOVA, so we are stuck with it. If we had kept it simple and stuck to the two products in which we were really interested, we might have been alright.

🔑 Do not elaborate experiments unnecessarily

Do not add in extra levels to experiments where there is no real need. You may dilute out a potentially detectable effect to the point where it is no longer statistically significant.

13.6 Chapter summary

A 'Factor' is an aspect of an experiment that we can alter to see if this changes the endpoint we are measuring. The various different possibilities for each factor are then referred to as 'levels'. While *t*-tests are used with the simplest experimental designs – a single experimental factor that has just two levels – for more complex designs, analyses of variance (ANOVAs) are called for.

   The one-way analysis of variance is used where there is a single factor that will be set to three or more levels. It is not appropriate to analyse such data by repeated *t*-tests as this will raise the risk of false positives above the acceptable level of 5 per cent. If the ANOVA produces a significant result, this only tells us that at least one level produces a different result from one of the others. It does not tell us which level differs from which other, nor does it tell us anything about the extent of the difference in the endpoint.

'Follow-up' tests will rectify both of these short-comings. Tukey's test will look at the difference for every possible pair of levels of the factor. Dunnett's test will treat one level as a reference and then compare all other levels against that. A confidence interval is calculated for the difference between each pair of treatments. If the interval excludes zero, that comparison is statistically significant The intervals are calculated to give each comparison less than a 5 per cent risk of producing a false positive. In this way, the entire series of comparisons will accumulate a total 5 per cent risk.

The two-way analysis of variance is used where two factors are being varied and all combinations of both factors have been studied. This ANOVA will test whether certain levels of each factor are consistently associated with high or low values for the endpoint. It will also test whether the effect of changing from one level to another within a factor is a constant increase/decrease or whether the effect seen depends upon the level of the other factor ('interaction'). Where interaction is present, a graphical method can be used to clarify what form the interaction takes.

More complex experiments (where three or more factors are varied) are possible and can be analysed by multi-way ANOVAs. However, such experiments can produce an unmanageable proliferation of combinations of treatments. Expert advice should be sought at an early stage.

ANOVAs allow the analysis of experiments of almost limitless complexity. It is important not to indulge in complexity for its own sake. Experimental design should be limited to the minimum that is required to answer your question. The inclusion of superfluous levels may dilute the effect you need to observe and render it non-significant.

14

Correlation and regression – relationships between measured values

This chapter will . . .

- Describe positive and negative correlation

- Show how the correlation coefficient (r) indicates both the nature and strength of any correlation between measured variables

- Describe how to test the statistical significance of correlation

- Emphasize that correlation is not necessarily proof of a cause and effect relationship

- Describe the use of regression equations to predict the value of a dependent variable ('response') from that of an independent one ('predictor')

- Warn against the casual use of extrapolation

- Demonstrate the 'reverse calculation' of the independent from the dependent variable

Essential Statistics for the Pharmaceutical Sciences   Philip Rowe
© 2007 John Wiley & Sons, Ltd   ISBN 9780 470 03470 5 (HB)   ISBN 9780 470 03468 2 (PB)

- Show how several predictors can be combined to estimate the value of a response, using multiple regression

- Describe the selection of a set of statistically significant predictors from a larger set of candidates

14.1 Correlation analysis

In this chapter we will be looking at interrelationships among measured variables. The simplest question is whether there is a relationship between two sets of measurements and, if so, how strong is that relationship. It is these questions that can be answered by correlation analysis.

The general concept of correlation is familiar enough. Age and handgrip strength are both variables that can be measured on appropriate interval scales (one in years and the other in Newtons). We are also sadly aware that, beyond a certain point, the inexorable increase in one value (age) is generally accompanied by an equally depressing decline in the other. It is this linkage between two measures that we recognize as correlation. Correlation does not require the linkage to be perfect, There will always be the odd 70-year-old with a grip to match or beat most 30-somethings, but there is a clear general trend.

14.1.1 Positive and negative correlation

In the example quoted above, increases in one parameter were associated with decreases in the other. We refer to this as 'negative correlation'. The term 'negative' should not be taken to imply an absence of correlation; it is just a particular form of correlation. In the contrasting situation, where both parameters tend to increase together, we refer to 'positive correlation'.

⚞ Positive and negative correlation

Positive – as one value increases the other also tends to increase.
Negative – as one value increases the other tends to decrease.

14.1.2 The correlation coefficient (*r*)

Instances of correlation vary in strength. The standardization graph for a colorimetric analytical method should show a very strong relationship between the

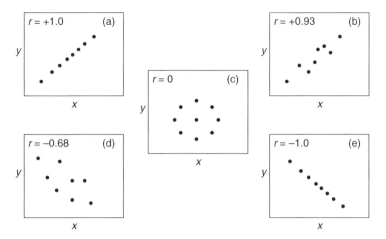

Figure 14.1 Information conveyed by the correlation coefficient (r)

measured absorption and the amount of analyte present. In contrast, in biological systems, where multiple factors tend to be at work, relationships are usually much vaguer. A graph of handgrip strength vs age would undoubtedly contain some pretty scattered points. The direction and strength of any correlation can be described by a statistic called the 'correlation coefficient'. For reasons that escape the author, this is given the symbol 'r'. (Note that a lower case r is used.)

The correlation coefficient can take any value between -1 and $+1$. Figure 14.1 shows examples of various types and strengths of correlation and the associated value of r. In this figure, the axes are simply labelled as x and y, so the graphs are general in nature. Parts (a) and (b) both show positive correlation, so r takes a positive value. In (d) and (e) negative correlation leads to negative values of r. In (c), there is no relationship and r is exactly zero. Cases (a) and (e) represent the most extreme forms of correlation – either perfect positive or perfect negative correlation. The associated r values are therefore also the most extreme values ($+1$ and -1). Cases (b) and (d) show partial correlation and the r values reflect the stronger correlation in (b) than in (d).

⚷ Correlation coefficient (r)

Describes the type and strength of correlation. It can take any value between -1 and $+1$

The correlation described in this chapter is 'Pearson correlation'. An alternative ('Spearman correlation') is described in Chapter 17. Pearson correlation is used so frequently that it is common to see it referred to simply as 'correlation'.

14.1.3 The need for significance testing of correlation coefficients

Imagine what would happen if two human characteristics were completely unre-
lated and we took a random selection of people and measured both characteristics
in each person. In an ideal world, we would get a set of results that yielded a
perfectly symmetrical graph like that seen in Figure 14.1(c) and an associated r
value of exactly zero. However in the real world, the points will almost always
show some slight upward or downward trend and the r value (whilst close to zero)
will take a small positive or negative value. Finding a degree of correlation within a
sample is not adequate justification for concluding that there must be correlation
in the wider population. We need to go through the usual approach of setting up a
null hypothesis and then assessing whether the evidence is consistent with such an
hypothesis.

🔑 Null and alternative hypotheses

Null – within the general population, the correlation coefficient between the two
   parameters is zero, i.e. they are uncorrelated.
Alternative – within the general population the correlation coefficient is non-zero, i.e.
   there is correlation of some type.

The null hypothesis assumes that, if some apparent correlation is present in the
sample, it arose by the mechanism shown in Figure 14.2. The underlying population
may be distributed perfectly symmetrically, with no correlation at all, but the random
sampling procedure must have selected points that create an impression of correlation (negative correlation in the example illustrated).

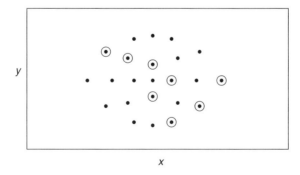

• Not selected for inclusion in the sample

⊙ Selected for inclusion in the sample

Figure 14.2 Mechanism assumed by null hypothesis when testing for correlation

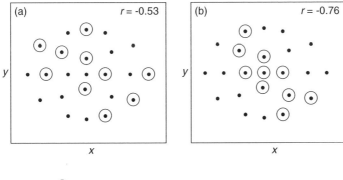

⊙ Observed value

• Hypothetical member of underlying population

Figure 14.3   Influence of the size of the correlation coefficient on the outcome of significance testing

14.1.4 Factors that will influence the outcome of significance testing

There are two factors that will be taken into account when testing this null
hypothesis – the size of the correlation coefficient and the sample size.

Size of the correlation coefficient   Figure 14.3(a) shows a sample with weak
correlation and also indicates a hypothetical, uncorrelated population from
which it might have been drawn. It is not difficult to imagine that random
sampling could quite easily lead to the vague appearance of correlation that we
see in part (a). In that case we would have to accept that the null hypothesis is
credible and there is inadequate evidence of correlation. However, in part (b) it
would be much less likely that we would randomly select this more strongly
correlated sample from an uncorrelated population. The null hypothesis becomes
difficult to believe and these data do provide significant evidence of correlation.
Note that the likelihood of significance depends upon what is called the 'absolute'
value of the correlation coefficient. The closer r is to either -1 or $+1$, the greater
the chances of significance; it is values around zero that are unlikely to prove
anything.

Sample size   Hopefully, the reader has by now twigged that the amount of data is an
issue in all significance tests. Correlation testing is no exception. In Figure 14.4(a), the
data points are well aligned and the correlation coefficient would be quite high, but
the null hypothesis is still perfectly credible – three randomly chosen points will quite
frequently form something approaching a straight line, but when 10 points all
confirm the same trend, as in Figure 14.4 (b), it is far more convincing.

Figure 14.5 summarizes the situation. As usual, the various factors can be offset
against each other. Therefore, for example, even very weak correlation can be

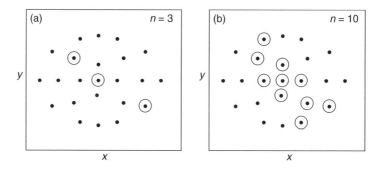

⊙ Observed value
• Hypothetical member of underlying population

Figure 14.4 Influence of sample size on the outcome of significance testing

statistically significant if enough observations are available. In contrast, small samples will only yield a significant outcome if correlation is very strong.

14.1.5 An example – drug content in leaves and the height at which the leaves grew

We are planning the commercial collection of the leaves of a species of tree from which a drug will be extracted. One question we need to consider is whether it is worth using ladders to gain access to leaves at the tops of the trees or whether we would be better just collecting the easily accessed, low growing leaves and moving on to the next tree. If the leaves at the tops of the trees were a markedly richer source of the drug that those lower down, then the use of ladders might be worthwhile, but otherwise we would prefer to stay on *terra firma*.

We therefore collect a trial series of 24 leaves, recording the heights at which they were growing on the tree and also analyse them for drug content. The results are shown in Table 14.1

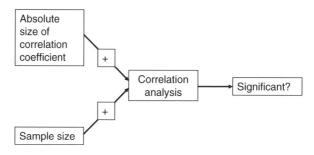

Figure 14.5 Factors influencing the outcome of significance testing for correlation

Table 14.1 Heights at which leaves were growing in the trees (m) and drug content (mg/100 g dry leaf)

Height (m)	Drug concentration (mg/100 g)	Height (m)	Drug concentration (mg/100 g)
1.70	1.66	3.23	1.27
2.31	1.34	3.29	0.85
2.89	1.27	3.46	1.16
1.30	1.61	3.95	1.14
3.21	1.17	1.70	1.25
1.84	1.73	2.92	1.49
3.27	1.17	2.67	1.17
4.21	1.19	3.02	1.16
1.32	1.93	2.37	1.75
3.67	1.10	2.64	1.36
2.78	1.37	4.25	1.00
3.71	1.19	1.90	1.48

14.1.6 Preliminary check for nonlinearity

Using statistical packages to perform correlation analysis is so simple that it is tempting to wade straight in. Be advised – do not. Correlation analysis is a search for a straight line relationship. The danger is that two sets of data may be strongly related but in a nonlinear manner. If a nonlinear relationship is present, correlation analysis can be very misleading. It is vital that you always inspect a simple graph of the data before proceeding to a statistical analysis. When we inspect the graph, we just need to satisfy ourselves that it does not provide unmistakable evidence of non-linearity. Figure 14.6 shows the types of patterns that are and are not acceptable. Parts

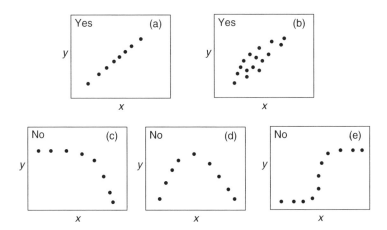

Figure 14.6 Is correlation analysis appropriate?

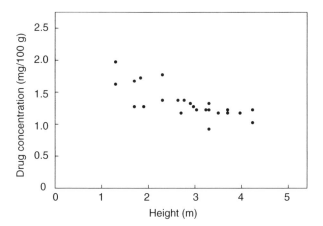

Figure 14.7 Drug concentration vs heights at which leaves were growing

(a) and (b) contain patterns where correlation analysis would be perfectly appropriate. Parts (c)–(e) show clear evidence of strongly nonlinear relationships and correlation analyses would produce misleading results.

The leaf data (Figure 14.7) show a pattern that could well be linear in nature and there is no objection to calculating a correlation coefficient.

⊸◯ Graphical inspection of the data

Data should be subjected to graphical inspection for any strong evidence of non-linearity before launching into a formal correlation analysis.

14.1.7 Performing correlation analysis

The two sets of data are invariably entered into two columns and then we merely identify the columns to be analysed. The output will include the correlation coefficient and a P value. Generic output for the height and drug content data would be as in Table 14.2. The r value is given as -0.777. The minus sign indicates negative correlation and a value of -0.777 tells us that there is quite a strong relationship. The results are also statistically significant ($P < 0.001$).

Table 14.2 Generic output for correlation analysis of height at which leaves were collected (m) and their drug content (mg/100 g)

Correlation analysis

Correlation of height and drug: $r = -0.777$
$P = 0.000$

The practical conclusion is pretty obvious. There is certainly no evidence that the higher leaves contain extra drug that might lead us to risk life and limb up a ladder. Indeed there is statistically significant evidence of quite the opposite pattern. We will stick to the nice easy leaves at the bottom, thank you very much!

14.1.8 A demonstration of correlation should not be assumed to imply a cause and effect relationship

The following data were obtained from the web site of the UK Government's Office of National Statistics (www.statistics.gov.uk):

- the percentage of UK households owning a microwave oven (data available for 7 years in the range 1991–2001);

- numbers of deaths from liver disease (deaths per million population) for the same years.

A graph of this data shows a very strong (and certainly statistically significant) association between the two (Figure 14.8).

Rising microwave use is associated with rising deaths from liver disease. How one would interpret this trend depends very much on what has gone before. If you have been exposed to a prolonged assertion that microwaves can interact detrimentally with liver cells, then you might be persuaded to start avoiding regular TV dinners. However, under more neutral circumstances, you would probably recognize that the points simply represent two independent time trends. The points on the graph are precisely in time order (left point = 1991, right = 2001). The graph then takes on its striking shape because during that decade there was a steady increase in microwave ownership (as with most consumer durables) and there was also a steady increase in fatal liver diseases. The reason for the rise in

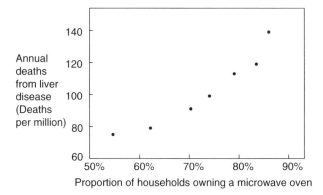

Figure 14.8 Microwave ovens and fatal liver diseases

such deaths is not immediately apparent, but there is absolutely no reason to attribute it to microwave ovens. The decade saw changes in all manner of social habits, exposure to novel chemicals and drugs, increased foreign travel and goodness knows what else, any of which could be the real cause of the increased mortality.

In this case the disjunction between correlation and a causal relationship is fairly obvious, but the general principal that you can have correlation without a cause and effect relationship always needs to be borne in mind. The greatest danger arises in those cases where a causal relationship seems feasible.

💀 💀 Plant the suggestion and then produce ☠ ☠ the pretty graph

The secret with this one, is doing things in the right order:

1. argue some sort of theoretical case that A would cause B; then

2. point out that if you are right then A and B ought to be correlated; and finally

3. produce the graph complete with impressive correlation. Naturally you will include a formal statistical analysis which will make it all look nice and official and nobody will argue.

Whether you get away with it depends largely on how effectively you complete stage 1. If that is done well, the overall effect can be highly seductive.

14.2 Regression analysis

14.2.1 An equation linking two measured variables

Correlation analysis only asks *whether* there is a relationship between two sets of data. Regression goes a step further and asks *how* are they related? More specifically it derives a mathematical equation that will allow us to predict one of the parameters if we know the value of the other.

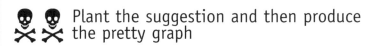 Regression analysis

Regression analysis produces an equation by which the value of the *dependent* variable can be predicted from the *independent* variable.

The box above emphasizes the fact that the equation operates in a specific direction. In order to undertake regression analysis, we have to decide which is the dependent and which the independent variable.

14.2.2 An example of regression – fungal toxin contamination and rainfall

To illustrate regression, we will consider another data set, also from the natural products arena. A drug precursor molecule is extracted from a type of nut. The nuts are commonly contaminated by a fungal toxin that is difficult to remove during the purification process. We suspect that the amount of fungus (and hence toxin) depends on rainfall at the growing site. We would like to be able to predict toxin concentration from rainfall in order to judge whether it would be worth paying additional rental charges for relatively drier sites. We analyse the toxin content in a series of batches of nuts and we also know the rainfall at the growing sites during the 4 months when the nuts are forming. The results are shown in Table 14.3. As with correlation, the first job is to check for any obvious nonlinearity in the data. Figure 14.9 shows that this is not a problem.

14.2.3 Identifying the line of best fit for the data – the least squares fit

We then want to find the best fitting straight line for the data. A possible line is shown in Figure 14.9. To determine how good a fit this line achieves, we determine the vertical distance (deviation) between each data point and the line. For example, the point corresponding to the lowest rainfall (0.51 cm/week) deviates very slightly

Table 14.3 Rainfall at the growing site and concentration of fungal toxin in nuts

Rain fall (cm/week)	Toxin (μg/100 g)
1.30	18.1
2.28	28.6
1.11	15.9
0.74	19.2
1.32	19.3
0.51	14.8
1.56	21.7
1.32	16.5
2.05	23.8
1.37	19.0

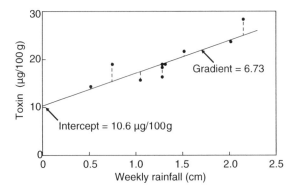

Figure 14.9 Regression line for fungal toxin and rainfall at growing site

above the line, the next point is further above and the next deviates below the line and so on. The broken vertical lines indicate the deviation for each point. We then square each of these individual deviations and add them up. This provides what is referred to as the 'sum of squares'. The sum of squares acts as an inverse measure of goodness of fit – the lower the value, the better the fit.

🔑 Sum of squares and the 'least squares fit'

Take all the vertical deviations of the points from the proposed line, square them and add them up. The lower the sum of squares, the better the fit. Select a line according to the 'least squares fit'.

The line of best fit is then the one with the lowest sum of squares. (The 'least squares fit') Fortunately we do not have to try endless different lines until we find the best. The line of best fit can be determined in a one-stage calculation.

14.2.4 The line of best fit and the regression equation

The line shown in Figure 14.9 is in fact the line of best fit. It intercepts the vertical axis at a value of 10.6 μg/100 g and it has a gradient of +6.73 (i.e. an increase in rainfall of 1 cm/week is associated with an increase in toxin concentration of 6.73 μg/100 g). Therefore, the line corresponds to the relationship:

$$\text{Toxin concentration } (\mu g/100\,g) = 10.6 + 6.73 \times \text{rainfall}$$

This is referred to as the regression equation.

14.2.5 Performing a regression analysis using a statistical package

The rainfall and toxin data will be entered into two appropriately labelled columns. You will then have to indicate the relevant columns. However, there is an important difference from correlation. With regression you must be careful to indicate correctly which is the dependent and which the independent variable. Unfortunately, statistical packages use a varied terminology. The toxin concentrations may be entered as the 'dependent variable' or 'response' and the rainfall may be the 'independent variable' or the 'predictor'.

Generic output is shown in Table 14.4. The order in which the various parts appear depends upon the particular statistical package. The first line tells us that the regression equation is:

$$\text{Toxin concentration} \ (\mu g/100\,g) = 10.6 + 6.73 \times \text{rainfall} \ (cm/week)$$

Regression analyses then traditionally produce a value called R-squared. This is in fact the square of the r value that we would get from a correlation analysis of the same data (expressed as a percentage). Like r, it gives a measure of how closely the points fit to a straight line. Zero indicates random scatter and 100 per cent a perfect fit to a straight line. The only problem is that the regression equation is supposed to be able to *predict* toxin from rainfall and none of this is true prediction. What we have done is to force a line to fit as tightly as possible to a known set of points. Any further data we acquire later will probably not fit the same line quite so well. Consequently, a slightly reduced value, 'R-squared adjusted' (0.724 or 72.4 per cent) is provided and is generally considered fairer. An R-squared of 72.4 per cent indicates that rainfall is a pretty good predictor of toxin.

Table 14.4 Generic output for regression analysis of toxin concentration and rainfall

Regression analysis

Regression equation: toxin $= 10.6 + 6.73 \times$ rainfall
R-Square $= 75.5\%$ R-Square (adjusted) $= 72.4\%$

Analysis of overall equation

Source	DF	SS	MS	F	P
Regression	1	114.84	114.84	24.61	0.001
Residual error	8	37.33	4.67		
Total	9	152.17			

Analysis of individual predictors

Predictor	Coefficient	SE coefficient	T	P
Constant	10.6	1.961	5.39	0.001
Rainfall	6.73	1.356	4.96	0.001

A lot of the output is concerned with the statistical significance of the regression equation. The null hypothesis is that, within the general population, there is actually no relationship between these two variables. This is essentially the same null hypothesis considered in correlation analysis. It is therefore no surprise that if a data set is subjected to both correlation and regression analyses the result is always the same. Either both analyses indicate significance or both non-significance – they never disagree. If you look at the next part of the output labelled 'analysis of overall equation', there is a *P* value of 0.001, which is strongly significant.

There will also be an analysis of the significance of the predictor. With simple regression, this part of the output adds nothing of value.

14.2.6   Making predictions using the regression equation

Having obtained the regression equation, we might now have the chance to rent two agricultural locations where we could grow a crop of nuts. Enquiries show that the weekly rainfall at sites A and B during the fruiting season are 2.05 and 1.25 cm/week, respectively. We could therefore predict that nuts grown at these two sites would contain:

Site A

$$\text{Toxin} = 10.6 + 6.73 \times \text{rainfall}$$
$$= 10.6 + 6.73 \times 2.05$$
$$= 10.6 + 13.8$$
$$= 24.4 \, \mu g/100 \, g$$

Site B

$$\text{Toxin} = 10.6 + 6.73 \times \text{rainfall}$$
$$= 10.6 + 6.73 \times 1.25$$
$$= 10.6 + 8.4$$
$$= 19.0 \, \mu g/100 \, g$$

With its lower rainfall, site B is predicted to produce a slightly better crop (22 per cent lower toxin load), but this modest advantage would have to be weighed against any cost differences between the two sites.

14.2.7   Extrapolation

Using the regression equation we could predict that, in an area with zero rainfall, nuts would contain $10.6 + 6.73 \times 0 = 10.6 \, \mu g/100 \, g$. However, this is clearly non-sense. In an arid desert . . . no trees . . . no nuts . . . no toxin . . . no nothing. We have direct evidence of a reasonably linear relationship between toxin and rainfall over an observed range of $0.51 - 2.28$ cm of rain per week. It is therefore reasonably safe to

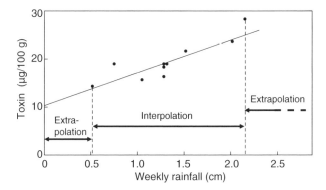

Figure 14.10 Interpolation and extrapolation

make predictions for any other site that has a rainfall figure within this range. This is referred to as 'interpolation'; see Figure 14.10.

As soon as we move outside this range, we have no knowledge of whether the straight line relationship continues. In reality it is unlikely that it does. In the Atacama Desert, the trees would simply die and in Cherapunjee (rain in excess of 100 cm a week) they would get washed away. Attempts to make predictions in cases where the value of the independent variable is outside the range we have actually observed are referred to as extrapolation. The general rule is that extrapolation should be avoided unless there is a sound theoretical reason to believe that the linear relationship continues beyond the observed range. In reality that is rarely the case, although some instances do arise. An example of reasonable extrapolation is carbon[14] dating. Nobody has ever observed C^{14} decaying for 5000 years, but once we have observed its behaviour for a couple of years, it is safe to predict its fate for the extra 4998 years.

Interpolation and extrapolation

Interpolation – a prediction using a value of the independent variable that is within the observed range; this is uncontroversial.

Extrapolation – a prediction using a value of the independent variable that lies outside the observed range. Extrapolation should be avoided unless there is sound reason to believe that the linear relationship extends beyond the observed range.

14.2.8 Reverse calculation

The normal purpose of regression is to be able to obtain a value for the dependent variable from the independent variable. However, there are times when we want to operate in the opposite direction. Classic examples are analytical methods that use a

Table 14.5 Quantity of PABA and resultant absorption at 510 nm

PABA (µg)	Absorption
0	0.00
5	0.11
5	0.10
10	0.20
10	0.20
15	0.30
15	0.32
20	0.41
20	0.40
25	0.50
25	0.51

calibration graph. For example, in a colorimetric method, we start with a set of standards and we can calculate a regression equation relating light absorption to amount of analyte in the usual way. However, in the next stage we will obtain readings of absorption for our unknown samples and will want to calculate their analyte contents. In that latter stage we are working backwards – calculating the independent variable (analyte concentration) from the dependent variable (absorption). The example below shows how this done.

Para-amino benzoic acid (PABA) can be measured by a diazotization reaction that yields a bright pink colour. The absorption is then measured at 510 nm. A series of standards yielded the results shown in Table 14.5. A graph of this data (Figure 14.11)

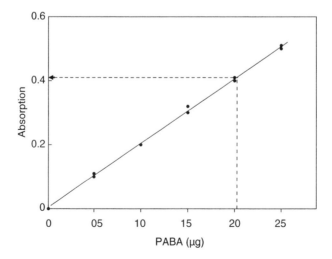

Figure 14.11 Reverse prediction of PABA concentration from absorption in a colorimetric analysis

shows excellent linearity, so regression analysis is appropriate. The regression analysis should treat the PABA concentration as the independent variable and absorption as the dependent. The regression equation is:

$$\text{Absorption} = 0.0023 + 0.0202 \times \text{PABA (µg)}$$

We can then re-arrange the equation so that it does what we want – allow us to calculate the PABA concentration from absorption.

$$\text{PABA (µg)} = \frac{\text{Absorption} - 0.0023}{0.0202}$$

If we then have an unknown sample with an absorption of (say) 0.41, its PABA content must be:

$$\text{PABA} = \frac{0.41 - 0.0023}{0.0202}$$

$$\text{PABA} = \frac{0.4077}{0.0202} \, \text{µg}$$

$$\text{PABA} = 20.2 \, \text{µg}$$

The procedure above seems rather cumbersome. Would it not be possible simply to carry out the regression, reversing the dependent and independent variables and get directly to an equation that predicts PABA concentration from absorption? We could do this, but the fitted line would be slightly different and would not be properly optimized. The correct procedure is the one shown above.

⚷ Reverse calculation

To predict the value of the independent from the dependent variable, the normal equation (predicting dependent from independent) is calculated initially and is then re-arranged.

14.3 Multiple regression

14.3.1 Using several predictors simultaneously

Multiple regression is a fairly complex subject with a number of potential pit-falls. This section is really only meant to give a taste of what it does. If you want to use it yourself, it would probably be a good idea to get some advice from a competent statistician.

In the previous example we used rainfall to predict toxin concentrations in crops of nuts. However, there may well be other aspects of the growing site that influence fungal growth. For example, sunshine and wind might tend to dry the trees and reduce fungal growth. We could set up a whole series of regression equations, each using one aspect of the growing site to make our predictions. However, each of these would be imprecise because if it used (say) wind speed then it would be ignoring the influence of rainfall and vice versa. What we want is a single equation that contains terms that reflect the influence of each relevant factor. The original regression equation contained a constant (a) and a term reflecting the influence of rainfall ($b \times$ rainfall):

$$\text{Predicted toxin concentration} = a + (b \times \text{Rainfall})$$

The term b is referred to as a 'coefficient'. There was a positive relationship between rainfall and toxin, so the value of coefficient b was positive. In that way the greater the rainfall, the greater the predicted toxin concentration.

To make use of several predictors simultaneously, all we do is add extra terms to cover each of the additional factors. If we have information about rainfall, temperature, daily hours of sunshine and wind speeds, the equation becomes:

$$\text{Predicted toxin concentration} = a + (b \times \text{rainfall}) + (c \times \text{temperature})$$
$$+ (d \times \text{sunshine}) + (e \times \text{wind})$$

We know that rainfall is positively related to toxin, but some of the other factors may show a negative relationship. For example, we might suspect that higher wind velocities would cause drying and lower fungal growth. This can be accommodated simply by giving the various coefficients (b–e) positive or negative values as appropriate.

⌫ Multiple regression

Multiple regression allows the prediction of a measured outcome, using several predictors. A regression equation is developed containing a separate term for each predictor. These terms consists of a coefficient multiplied by the value of the particular predictor.

14.3.2 An example – using several meteorological variables to predict fungal toxin levels

Table 14.6 shows the same data as Table 14.2, but also includes the additional data concerning temperature, sunshine and wind.

Table 14.6 Rainfall, temperature, sunshine and wind speed at growing sites and concentration of fungal toxin in nuts

Rain (cm/week)	Noon temperature (°C)	Sunshine (h/day)	Wind speed (km/h)	Toxin (µg /100 g)
1.30	20.9	6.23	13.3	18.1
2.28	25.4	8.13	10.8	28.6
1.11	28.2	10.21	10.9	15.9
0.74	23.7	6.96	8.2	19.2
1.32	26.5	9.04	9.8	19.3
0.51	23.9	7.84	12.3	14.8
1.56	26.7	6.69	10.0	21.7
1.32	30.0	8.30	12.2	16.5
2.05	24.9	9.22	10.7	23.8
1.37	22.0	8.37	15.0	19.0

14.3.3 Performing multiple regression

Start with all the potential predictors In a statistical package, the data are entered into five columns and then you will have to indicate that toxin is the dependent variable/response and the four meteorological factors the independent variables/predictors. Generic output is shown in Table 14.7.

The first thing to notice (under 'analysis of overall equation') is that the regression equation is statistically significant ($P = 0.006$). However, all this tells us is that the

Table 14.7 Generic output for regression analysis of toxin concentration with all potential predictors (rainfall, temperature, sunshine and wind)

Regression analysis

Regression equation:

Toxin $= 31.6 + 7.07 \times$ rain $- 0.420 \times$ temperature $- 0.237 \times$ sun $- 0.794 \times$ wind
R-squared $= 91.9\%$ R-squared (adjusted) $= 85.3\%$

Analysis of overall equation

Source	DF	SS	MS	F	P
Regression	4	139.782	34.946	14.11	0.006
Residual error	5	12.387	2.477		
Total	9	152.169			

Analysis of individual predictors

Predictor	Coefficient	SE coefficient	T	P
Constant	31.6	7.105	4.45	0.007
Rain	7.07	1.003	7.05	0.001
Temperature	−0.420	0.2413	−1.74	0.142
Sun	−0.237	0.5086	−0.47	0.660
Wind	−0.794	0.2977	−2.67	0.045

equation as a whole probably does have real predictive power. The problem is that the effectiveness of the equation might be due solely to the fact that it takes rainfall into account (which we already know to be a useful predictor.) It is possible that some (or all) of the other factors we have added may be doing nothing to improve the accuracy of prediction. To test this we need to look at the section 'analysis of individual predictors'. Here we find P values for each individual predictor. Rain and wind are shown with P values of 0.001 and 0.045, so both are significant. The other two (temperature and sunshine) are apparently not significant.

Remove non-significant variables one at a time   What we now need to do is start removing the non-significant factors from the regression equation. However, we do not immediately reject both temperature and sunshine. Multiple regression behaves rather strangely if two of the predictors are themselves correlated. In this case temperature and sunshine are (not surprisingly) positively correlated. (The r value is +0.501) This means that there is an element of redundancy – the two sets of values largely reflect the same information. Consequently, it may well be true that we do not need to retain both factors. Unfortunately, when multiple regression analysis encounters two factors that are markedly correlated it tends to report that we do not need either! The correct way to proceed is to eliminate one of these factors and see what happens to the other. We will either find that the remaining factor is now miraculously revealed as significant (in which case we obviously retain it) or it will remain non-significant and we can get rid of it as well. The remaining question is which we should remove first – temperature or sunshine? From a purely statistical point of view, we would prefer to retain the factor that is closest to significance. Since temperature had a P value of 0.142 it has a stronger claim to be retained than sunshine ($P = 0.660$). In the absence of any other consideration we would probably drop sunshine and try again. Occasionally our knowledge of the particular situation may lead us to believe that some factor is of special importance and ought to be retained. This might then over-ride purely statistical considerations. In this case, there is no such special knowledge and we will repeat the regression, using rainfall, temperature and wind, but omitting sunshine. The output is now as in Table 14.8.

We now have the happy situation that the equation as a whole is significant ($P = 0.001$), and all the contributory factors (rain, temperature and wind) have significant P values (<0.001, 0.047 and 0.023, respectively).

🔑 Removing non-significant factors from multiple regression equations

When two or more factors are shown to be apparently non-significant, do *not* remove them all simultaneously. Remove one factor at a time until all the remaining factors are statistically significant.

Table 14.8 Generic output for regression analysis of toxin concentration with sunshine removed, leaving rainfall, temperature and wind as predictors

Regression analysis

Regression equation:

Toxin $= 31.6 + 7.01 \times$ rain $- 0.479 \times$ temperature $- 0.822 \times$ wind
R-squared $= 91.5\%$ R-squared (adjusted) $= 87.3\%$

Analysis of overall equation

Source	DF	SS	MS	F	P
Regression	3	139.242	46.414	21.54	0.001
Residual error	6	12.927	2.155		
Total	9	152.169			

Predictor	Coef	SE coefficient	T	P
Constant	31.6	6.625	4.76	0.003
Rain	7.01	0.9285	7.55	0.000
Temperature	−0.479	0.1919	−2.50	0.047
Wind	−0.822	0.2718	−3.02	0.023

14.3.4 The final equation

The regression equation is:

Toxin concentration $= 31.6 + (7.01 \times$ rain$) - (0.479 \times$ temperature$) - (0.822 \times$ wind$)$

The term for rainfall still has a plus sign, so higher rainfall will increase the predicted toxin concentrations. However, temperature and wind speed have minus signs, so high temperatures and strong winds are presumably associated with drying and lower toxin concentrations. Biologically, this is all perfectly reasonable.

14.3.5 Forward selection of variables

In Section 14.3.3 we selected our predictors by starting with the full set and eliminating those considered irrelevant ('reverse elimination'). It is possible to use 'forward selection' where you start by finding the best single predictor and then look for the best additional variable to accompany it and so on. At each stage, the significance of all predictors is tested and you stop when you can no longer find a further variable that could be added and would achieve statistical significance.

There is no absolute case for preferring either approach, but for selection among a limited number of potential predictors, the author has generally found reverse elimination satisfactory. The one situation where forward selection is nigh on unavoidable is where there are very large numbers of potential predictors. To undertake reverse elimination you might have to start with a regression equation containing 100 terms. (However, see the caution in Section 14.3.8 against trawling through excessive numbers of possible predictors.)

Table 14.9 Meteorological data for two potential growing sites

Site	Rain (cm/week)	Noon temperature (°C)	Wind speed (km/h)
A	2.05	26.1	11.0
B	1.25	22.5	9.1

14.3.6 Using the equation to predict toxin contamination

Let us return to the two potential sites that we already compared on the basis of rainfall alone, but now take account of temperature and wind speed as well. The fuller data for these two sites are shown in Table 14.9.

In our in initial prediction (based on rainfall alone), site B seemed better as it had a lower rainfall. However, we can now see that the other factors favour site A (higher temperatures and stronger winds). Taking everything into account, our predictions would now be:

Site A

$$\text{Toxin concentration} = 31.6 + (7.01 \times \text{rain}) - (0.479 \times \text{temperature}) - (0.822 \times \text{wind})$$
$$= 31.6 + (7.01 \times 2.05) - (0.479 \times 26.1) - (0.822 \times 11.0)$$
$$= 31.6 + 14.37 - 12.5 - 9.04$$
$$= 24.43 \, \mu g/100 g$$

Site B

$$\text{Toxin concentration} = 31.6 + (7.01 \times \text{rain}) - (0.479 \times \text{temperature}) - (0.822 \times \text{wind})$$
$$= 31.6 + (7.01 \times 1.25) - (0.479 \times 22.5) - (0.822 \times 9.1)$$
$$= 31.6 + 8.76 - 10.78 - 7.48$$
$$= 22.10 \, \mu g/100 g$$

The effects of higher temperatures and wind speeds at site A have not quite offset the effects of the lower rainfall at site B and the latter continues to be predicted to be the better site. However, the difference is now very small and we need to bear in mind that all these predictions are only approximate. There is effectively nothing to choose between the two sites.

14.3.7 Better fit with more predictors

The final output (Table 14.8) shows an adjusted R-squared value of 0.873, which is higher than the value of 0.724 achieved by simple regression using rainfall alone. The multiple regression equation would be expected to achieve better prediction of toxin concentration, as it takes account of more factors.

14.3.8 Multiple testing

In Chapter 13, it was emphasized that multiple t-tests were not acceptable as they constituted multiple testing and would increase the risk of false positives. Multiple regression inevitably brings with it a degree of multiple testing as we are considering several factors and running a 5 per cent risk of a false positive with each one. In the case studied above, we initially considered only four factors and three of these were retained as apparently significant, so it is unlikely that these were actually false positive findings. A further defence of our finding is that the three factors selected were all biologically plausible.

The real danger arises if we start with a large number of possible factors and insist on picking out a small number of these. For example, if we were trying to relate the biological activity of a series of molecules to their chemical properties (quantitative structure–activity relationships), we could use modern computer software to generate literally hundreds of chemical descriptors for the molecules in question. Let us assume that we start looking for relationships between all of these descriptors and the biological activities and let us also assume that none of the descriptors actually has the slightest relationship to the endpoint. By the time we have trawled through (say) 100 descriptors, 1 in 20 cases will generate false positives and we would expect to find several 'predictors', each carrying its own individual (and apparently comforting) P value of less than 0.05. We could then discard the 90+ descriptors that have been correctly identified as irrelevant and publish a multiple regression equation based on the handful of false positives.

When faced with any claim that a significant regression (or multiple regression) equation has been discovered, it is always worth asking how many potential predictors were initially considered.

 Check large numbers of possible 'predictors' and exploit the false positives

Some areas of research have been so bedevilled with this nonsense that you are unlikely to get away with it, but choose a virgin field and there may yet be some mileage.

What you need is a nice big data base, with lots of sets of values for factors that might be related to the matter in hand (you really need a minimum of 20 or 30 candidates). Trawl vigorously, rejecting 95 per cent of the factors as non-significant. Publish the remainder, placing great emphasis on those lovely low P values, which undoubtedly prove that this select band of flukes are genuine predictors.

14.4 Chapter summary

Correlation and regression analyses describe the relationships between measured variables (generally on interval scales). Correlation may be positive (values increase or decrease together) or negative (increases in one value associated with decreases in the other). The correlation coefficient describes what type of relationship exists (positive or negative) and the strength of the association. It may take any value between -1 and $+1$. Before calculating the correlation coefficient, a graphical check should be made for any clear evidence of a nonlinear relationship. The statistical significance of correlation will depend upon the value of the correlation coefficient and the number of observations. A demonstration of correlation should not automatically be assumed to provide evidence of a cause and effect relationship.

In regression analysis, we identify the best fitting straight line through the observed data points. This is selected on the basis that it minimizes the sum of the squared vertical deviations of the points from the line – the 'least squares fit'. The goodness of fit is reported as an R-squared value which can vary between 0 (no fit) and 100 per cent (perfect fit of line to points).

The equation of the regression line can then be used to predict the value of the dependent variable from that of the independent. This equation will take the form:

$$y = a + bx$$

where a represents the intercept of the regression line with the vertical axis and b (the coefficient) is the gradient of the line.

When computing the regression equation, it is vital to identify correctly which is the dependent and which the independent variable. Once a regression equation has been developed, it can be used to predict the value of the dependent variable for a new case, using the value of the independent variable. When making such predictions, values of the independent variable should be within the range of observed values that were used to create the regression equation (interpolation). The use of values outside the observed values (extrapolation) should be avoided unless there is good reason to believe that the linear relationships continues beyond the observed range. If it is necessary to estimate the value of the independent variable from the dependent (reverse prediction), the normal regression equation should be calculated initially and then algebraically re-arranged.

Regression can be extended to multiple regression, allowing several factors to participate in the prediction of the dependent variable. For every additional factor considered, an additional term is added to the regression equation shown above. It is necessary to establish not only that the equation is significant overall, but also that each individual contributing factor is significant. If some of the factors are found to be non-significant, these should be removed one at a time and significance re-tested at each stage, stopping once all remaining factors are individually significant. Readers should be wary of claims to have found significant regression equations, if the factors used in the equation are a small subset from a much larger initial collection; some (or all) of the factors claimed as statistically significant may be no more than false positives.

Part 3

Nominal-scale data

15

Describing categorized data

This chapter will ...

- Show how we describe nominal scale data (data that consist of categorizations rather than measurements)

- Describe the production of a 95 per cent confidence interval for a proportion

- Emphasise the inefficient nature of nominal scale data

- Describe the use of the goodness-of-fit chi-square test to determine whether the true proportion of a particular class of things/individuals might credibly be some pre-determined figure

In this chapter we will start to look at data where no measurements are made on individuals. Instead, each individual is placed in a category and the numbers in each category are then counted. A classic example is where we look at a medical treatment and declare each patient's outcome as 'successful' or 'unsuccessful'. We then count the number of successes and failures. This type of data was introduced in Chapter 1 as 'nominal' scale data.

Essential Statistics for the Pharmaceutical Sciences Philip Rowe
© 2007 John Wiley & Sons, Ltd   ISBN 9780 470 03470 5 (HB)   ISBN 9780 470 03468 2 (PB)

15.1 Descriptive statistics

15.1.1 Proportions in each category

To describe measurement data we needed indicators of both the overall magnitude of the values (mean, etc.) and their variability (SD). Describing nominal-type data is simpler because all we can report is the proportion of individuals falling into each category. Many categorizations form just two groups e.g. succeed/fail, alive/dead, male/female. This is referred to as a dichotomization and we usually call the proportions falling into each category p and q. Which category is allocated to p and which to q is completely arbitrary. For example if 50 patients receive a treatment and 42 were considered to have had a successful outcome (leaving eight unsuccessful), then we might allocate p and q so that:

Proportion successful $= (p) = 42/50 = 0.84$ or 84%
Proportion unsuccessful $= (q) = 8/50 = 0.16$ or 16%

We have already met P values in the context of significance testing and it is singularly unfortunate that the same letter should be introduced for a second important function, but then that is statistics for you. (To achieve some clarity. I will use lower case p for proportion and upper case P in hypothesis testing.)

15.1.2 What determines the precision of sample estimates of a proportion?

As with measurement data, we need to distinguish between sample and population proportions. The data we analyse will almost invariably be sample data collected in a survey or experiment which was intended to estimate the proportions within some wider population. The proportions derived from samples will rarely exactly match those in the underlying population. With this type of data, sampling error depends simply upon the number of observations. Figure 15.1 shows the pattern that emerged with repeated sampling from the same population of individuals, 50 per cent of whom respond successfully to a treatment and 50 per cent were treatment failures. Various different sample sizes were used. With samples as small as 10, there was wide scatter. Some samples contained only 2/10 successes while others contained 8/10, suggesting a success rate of anything between 20 and 80 per cent. Samples this small are just about useless. Even samples of 25 or 50 were often pretty misleading and we really needed samples of 100 or more before we got tolerably reliable estimates.

⚍○ Precision of an estimated proportion

The precision with which a proportion within the population can be estimated from a sample depends solely on the number counted. Greater numbers – greater precision.

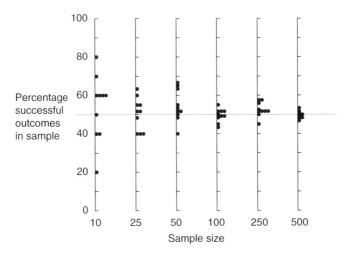

Figure 15.1 Ten estimates of the proportion of successful outcomes – various sample sizes (true proportion – 50 per cent)

15.1.3 The 95 per cent confidence intervals for a proportion

In the example quoted earlier, we found that 42 out of a sample of 50 patients (84 per cent) showed a successful response to treatment, but, what would happen if we were to adopt this treatment and record the outcomes for thousands of patients over the next few years? The proportion of successful outcomes would (hopefully) settle down to a figure in the region of 84 per cent, but it would be most surprising if our original sample provided an exact match to the long-term figure. To deal with this, we quote 95 per cent confidence intervals for the proportion in the population based upon a sample proportion.

15.1.4 Using a stats package to produce a 95 per cent confidence interval for a dichotomized proportion

Statistical packages differ in the way in which they expect data to be supplied. Some will only work from the raw data. For our success/fail data, you would provide the data as a column containing the 50 results coded suitable (possibly an 'S' or an 'F' for each success or failure).

Other packages will allow either the above format or 'summarized data'. In the latter case you indicate the total number of individuals examined and the number falling into one of the two available categories. (It is completely arbitrary which category you supply.)

In the generic output (Table 15.1) the data have been supplied in summarized form, indicating 50 cases examined and 42 classified as 'successes'.

Table 15.1 Generic output for calculation of a 95 per cent CI for the proportion of successes

95% CI for proportions	
Number examined	50
Number detected (successful)	42
Point estimate (successful)	84%
95% CI for proportion (successful)	70.9–92.8%

The 95 per cent confidence interval is 70.9–92.8 per cent, so the most we can say is that, if this therapy were implemented, we would expect the success rate to settle down eventually somewhere within the rather broad range of about 71–93 per cent.

15.1.5 Nominal data are not very efficient

With measurement data, we were often able to draw useful conclusions based on quite small numbers (10 or 15) of individuals. Here we have a somewhat larger sample (50) and yet the conclusion is horribly fuzzy, with a 95 per cent CI covering a range of nearly 22 percentage points. Unfortunately it is a characteristic of this type of data that you need to gather an awful lot of it before you achieve any worthwhile degree of precision. Figure 15.1 showed that, unless samples were quite large, they really were not very reliable. This should translate into the widths of 95 per cent CIs Figure 15.2 shows that this is indeed the case.

We have a series of samples of increasing size, each of which give a point estimate of 50 per cent for the success rate. Samples of 10 or 20 are almost useless, because the 95 per cent CIs are ridiculously wide. If our target for precision was a CI covering no more than 10 percentage points (which does not seem overly ambitious), we would need a sample size of almost 500.

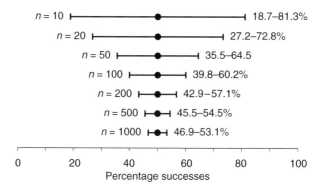

Figure 15.2 The 95 per cent confidence intervals for the proportion of successful outcomes to treatment with varying sample sizes

> 🔑 **Inefficiency of nominal scale data**
>
> You need to gather an awful lot of observations to achieve a useful degree of precision.

15.1.6 The other category

If you need a CI for the proportion in the other category (failures in the present case), it is fortunately just a case of subtracting the values we already obtained from 100 per cent. Thus the confidence limits for the proportion of failures would be 7.2–29.1 per cent

15.1.7 Ninety-five per cent CIs for proportions are generally asymmetrical

Figure 15.3 refers back to our trial where 42 out of 50 patients showed a successful outcome. Notice that the interval is asymmetrical. The asymmetry arises because possible values are more tightly constrained on one side than the other. The upper limit of the interval could not logically be greater than 100 per cent, so the upper limit cannot be far above the point estimate of 84 per cent. However, the lower limit could be anything down to 0 per cent. Confidence intervals for proportions are always asymmetrical, unless the point estimate happens to be exactly 50 per cent (as in Figure 15.2).

15.1.8 The problem of rare events

The inefficiency of nominal scale data is further exacerbated when one of the categories is rare. For example, a drug may produce a side-effect in a small proportion of users. In the example that follows, we will assume a 4 per cent occurrence rate. If we studied 500 patients that might sound like a perfectly adequate number.

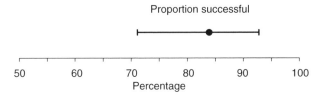

Figure 15.3 The 95 per cent confidence interval for the proportion of successful outcomes (42/50)

However, while that will produce plenty of individuals who are free of the side-effect (~480), we would only anticipate finding 20 who do suffer it – a quite inadequate number. What we have to ensure is that we detect an acceptable number of individuals in all categories. The problem in this case is to accumulate sufficient individuals who do suffer the side-effect. We know from previous examples that (as an absolute minimum) any category with less than 50–100 observations will yield only a very imprecise estimate of the proportion. So, with a 4 per cent occurrence rate, we would have to observe 1250 patients to find 50 with the side-effect. Even having checked out over 1000 people, if we take the figures of 50 cases out of 1250, the 95 per cent CI for the proportion with the side effect will be 2.98–5.24 per cent which is still not stunningly precise.

⛌ Rare events make matters even worse

If only a small proportion of individuals fall into one of the available categories, the number of observations required will escalate still further, because it will be hard to accumulate enough observations in the rare category.

15.2 Testing whether the population proportion might credibly be some pre-determined figure

15.2.1 Using the 95 CI for the proportion

Where individuals are being categorized into two groups, we could test a hypothesis that the proportion in one of the categories was some stated figure by inspecting the 95 per cent CI. For example, in the case of the condition being treated in Section 15.1.1, we might know that about 50 per cent of individuals will get better spontaneously and so a placebo will produce a 50 per cent success rate. Is the success rate with our treatment any different from what would have happened anyway? We would set up a null hypothesis that the true proportion of successes with our treatment is 50 per cent. If the figure of 50 per cent fell within the CI, the null hypothesis would remain credible. In fact it does not, so we have significant evidence that the true proportion of successes with our treatment is not 50 per cent. (Fortunately it is above rather than below the assumed placebo rate of success!)

15.2.2 The goodness-of-fit chi-square test

The above is a perfectly reputable approach, but we are going to introduce a separate test (goodness-of-fit chi-square test). There are two reasons for this:

1. The chi-square test is one of the oldest and most venerable statistical tests and you will certainly come across cases where other people have used it. You may also want to use it yourself as you know your readers are likely to be familiar with it.

2. The chi-square test is flexible (it can be applied in situations where cases are categorized into more than two classes).

'Chi' is a letter of the Greek alphabet and chi-square is often written as χ^2. This test is not implemented in all statistical packages, but is so simple to calculate that we can realistically perform it manually.

⊶◎ Goodness-of-fit chi-square test

Compares the proportion within a sample with some hypothesized proportion for the population. Is the sample data consistent with the specified proportion?

15.2.3 Goodness-of-fit chi-square test for two categories – returned pressurized canisters

The example we will consider in detail is a company that produces pressurized canisters of drug for asthma inhalers. Their factory has two machines that manufacture the canisters. One machine (Allegro model) is faster and produces 61 per cent of the factory's output. The slower machine (Andante model) produces the other 39 per cent. Occasional canisters are returned as faulty, and over the previous year, 126 of these have accumulated. From the batch numbers on the canisters we can determine that 52 were manufactured on the Allegro machine and 74 on the Andante. Since only a minority of canisters are made on the Andante machine, and yet it generates the majority of returns, we suspect that the output from this machine is less reliable. However, a formal statistical test is required.

First we need a null hypothesis. This will state that the products of the two machines are equivalent and if we went on collecting dodgy canisters for long enough the proportions of returns from each machine would simply be proportional to the numbers they produced. More formally it would be: 'among a large population of returned canisters 61 per cent would be from the Allegro machine and 39 per cent from the Andante'.

To perform the test we first calculate the so-called 'expected frequencies'. These are an idealized set of frequencies calculated to match the null hypothesis exactly. So with our 126 returned canisters, the null hypothesis claims that 61 per cent of these should be from the Allegro and 39 per cent from the Andante machine. Hence, the 'expected' frequencies are $126 \times 0.61 = 76.86$ (Allegro) and $126 \times 0.39 = 49.14$ (Andante). Notice that the term 'expected' is being used in a technical sense. There is no

Table 15.2   Calculation of the goodness-of-fit chi-square test

	Allegro	Andante
Observed	52	74
Expected	76.86	49.14
Observed – expected (discrepancy)	−24.86	+24.86
(Observed – expected)^2	618	618
(Observed – expected)^2/expected	8.04	12.58
χ^2		$8.04 + 12.58 = 20.62$

expectation, in the normal sense, that we would observe these precise figures in the real world (especially as they involve decimal places!). We then calculate the test as in Table 15.2.

> ## 🗝 'Expected frequencies'
>
> These are calculated so as to match exactly with the null hypothesis. There is no literal expectation that we would detect these numbers in a real world experiment.

The first two rows show the real observed figures and the so-called 'expected' frequencies that would have matched the null hypothesis exactly. The key line is the next one, which shows the discrepancies between what we observed and what the null hypothesis led us to expect. The negative number (-24.86) indicates that we observed fewer sub-standard canisters from the Allegro machine than we would have expected on the basis of the null hypothesis. The positive figure is the excess of canisters from the Andante machine. It is the size of these numbers that determines whether or not the outcome will be significant. Small discrepancies would indicate that the null hypothesis is in reasonable agreement with what we actually observed and is therefore acceptable. However, large discrepancies suggest that the null hypothesis was completely wrong and should be dismissed. It is this attempt to match up the observed and expected frequencies that leads to the test being called a 'goodness-of-fit' test.

The rest of the calculation is a classic statistical 'sausage machine'. In the next line the discrepancies are squared and then these are divided by the expected frequency. In the final line, we sum the last two figures to produce the test statistic $-\chi^2$. A large value for χ^2 would provide sufficient evidence that the null hypothesis is inconsistent with what was actually observed and should be dismissed. Exactly how big the χ^2 value has to be for the result to be statistically significant is shown in Table 15.3.

Notice that the required ('critical') value of χ^2 depends upon the number of categories that have been used. In this case, there were only two categories

Table 15.3   The χ^2 value required for a goodness-of-fit chi-square test to be statistically significant ($P < 0.05$)

Number of categories	Critical χ^2 value
2	3.842
3	5.991
4	7.815
5	9.488
6	11.070

(Allegro or Andante), so the critical χ^2 is 3.842. Our data set yielded a χ^2 of 20.62. As the value we achieved is way in excess of the critical value, our conclusion is very clearly significant. There is overwhelming evidence that the Andante machine is producing a disproportionately high proportion of the faulty canisters.

15.2.4 The 'continuity' problem

The mathematical basis of the test includes an assumption that the χ^2 values are 'continuous'. In other words, they could take any value. The reality, however, is that, when we count canisters (or any other set of discrete items), the results are 'discontinuous' – we may observe 1, 2 or 3 canisters, etc., but not a fractional value. The subsequent chi-square values are therefore also discontinuous – some values of χ^2 could never arise because they do not match any outcome based upon whole numbers of canisters. This mis-match between the assumptions made by the test and the reality of the data introduces a bias that may inflate the χ^2 value and make the data look a little more significant that it really is.

The most commonly advocated solution to this problem is the introduction of the Yates correction. However, the use of this correction is somewhat problematic as it is rather drastic and tends to overshoot, sometimes converting a liberal situation (too willing to declare significance) into a conservative one (too reluctant). We need a policy that never produces a markedly misleading result and is not so complex or obscure as to arouse suspicions that some sort of statistical fiddle is afoot. A simple and commonly used rule is that we should apply Yates correction only where there are just two categories. With more than two categories, the effect of discontinuity is so small, we are better off not trying to compensate for it.

As our problem with the canisters does have just two categories, the Yates correction should be added. The re-worked calculation, including the correction is shown in Table 15.4. The correction requires adjusting the discrepancies between the observed and expected frequencies by 0.5. The correction is applied so as to move the value towards zero. So a negative figure such as -24.86 is adjusted upwards to -24.36 whereas $+24.86$ moves down to $+24.36$.

Table 15.4 Calculation of the goodness-of-fit chi-square test with Yates correction

	Allegro	Andante
Observed	52	74
Expected	76.86	49.14
Observed – expected (discrepancy)	−24.86	+24.86
Observed – expected (Yates correction)	−24.36	+24.36
(Observed – expected)^2	593	593
(Observed – expected)^2/expected	7.72	12.07
χ^2	$7.72 + 12.07 = 19.79$	

⚿ Yates correction

Apply the correction only when there are just two categories. Correct the discrepancies between observed and expected frequencies by 0.5, moving the value towards zero.

The effect of the correction depends on the magnitude of the data, only being noticeable with very small figures. The numbers involved here are quite modest, but are still big enough to make the effect of the correction minimal. The value of χ^2 is reduced from 20.62 to 19.79 and the result remains clearly significant.

15.2.5 Cases with more than two categories – patient preferences among three information leaflets

Dealing with cases where there are more than two categories is a simple extension of the method already shown. An example is given below.

A series of 90 patients are each shown three different leaflets explaining the proper use of an inhaler. They are all asked to identify which of the three they considered the easiest to read and understand. The patients have thereby grouped themselves into three categories according to their preference. We then want to test whether there is any significant evidence of differences among the acceptability of the leaflets. The numbers selecting each leaflet (A, B or C) are shown in Table 15.5:

There appears to be some preference for leaflet B, but we need a formal statistical test to see if the trend is significant. Our null hypothesis is that all leaflets are equally likely to be selected and so our 'expected' outcome is that each leaflet will be selected by $90/3 = 30$ patients. We then calculate χ^2 in the usual way (Table 15.6). Notice that Yates correction has not been applied as there are more than two categories. According to Table 15.3 (three categories), χ^2 would need to achieve a value of at

Table 15.5 Numbers of patients selecting a leaflet as their preference

Leaflet	Number of Patients
A	23
B	39
C	28

Table 15.6 Calculation of the goodness-of-fit chi-square test for patients preferring one of three leaflets

	Leaflet A	Leaflet B	Leaflet C
Observed	23	39	28
Expected	30	30	30
Observed − expected (discrepancy)	−7	+9	−2
(Observed − expected)^2	49	81	4
(Observed − expected)^2/expected	1.63	2.70	0.13
χ^2		$1.63 + 2.70 + 0.13 = 4.46$	

least 5.991 for the result to be statistically significant. So, at this stage, we have not positively demonstrated any differences among the leaflets.

Care is needed in deciding what practical action should be taken on the basis of this result. Remember that a non-significant result does not preclude a difference. Leaflet B has quite a strong lead over its competitors and our experiment may simply have inadequate power to detect a genuine superiority. This is another demonstration of how frustrating this type of data can be −90 patients recruited and interviewed and we still are not sure if it matters which leaflet we use!

15.3 Chapter summary

Categorization (nominal scale) data are dealt with using statistical methods entirely different from those previously encountered with measurement (interval scale) data. To describe such data, we report the proportion of individuals falling into each category. Sample data can be used to estimate the proportion of individuals falling into a given category in the general population, but this process is subject to random sampling error. The extent of sampling error depends only upon the numbers observed, with greater numbers giving greater precision. This type of data is rather inefficient. Large numbers need to be observed before any real precision is achieved and this problem is further exacerbated if one (or more) of the categories only contain a small proportion of individuals.

Where the data arise from a dichotomization, most statistical packages provide a routine to calculate a 95 per cent CI for the proportion of individuals in a category. Such CIs are asymmetrical (except where each category accounts for exactly 50 per cent of the sample).

The goodness-of-fit chi-square test can be used to determine whether the population proportion for any category might credibly be some pre-determined figure. The test can be applied to data arising from classification into any number of categories, but if only two categories are being considered, the Yates correction should be applied. The test is not implemented by all statistical packages, but is simple enough to allow manual calculation.

16

Comparing observed proportions – the contingency chi-square test

---

This chapter will . . .

- Describe contingency tables

- Show the use of the contingency chi-square test to detect changes in proportions under different circumstances

- Advocate the use of simple 2 × 2 tables wherever possible

- Show the use of a 95 per cent CI for the difference between two proportions to test for a practically significant difference

- Show how to determine necessary sample size for an experiment that is to be analysed by a contingency chi-square test

---

Essential Statistics for the Pharmaceutical Sciences   Philip Rowe
© 2007 John Wiley & Sons, Ltd   ISBN 9780 470 03470 5 (HB)   ISBN 9780 470 03468 2 (PB)

16.1 Using the contingency chi-square test to compare observed proportions

16.1.1 Expulsion rates of IUDs – an example of a contingency table

In this chapter, we want to compare the proportion of individuals who end up in a particular category under two (or more) differing circumstances. For example we might want to compare two groups of women using alternative designs of intra-uterine device (IUD). We want to see if there is any difference in the proportion of women for whom the IUD is accidentally expelled from the womb during the first 6 months of use. We randomly allocate 4000 women to two equal sized groups. One group is fitted with an existing (control) design and the other group all receive a new (test) design. After 6 months we follow up to determine the outcomes.

The results obtained can be expressed in a so-called contingency table as in Table16.1. The characteristic feature of a contingency table is that both the columns and rows are based on categorizations. Here, the columns are based on the category of IUD used and the rows are based on outcomes, which are also categorized.

☞ Contingency tables

A table where the columns and rows are based upon categorization.

Since both the columns and rows of a contingency table are formed on the basis of categorizations, the table could be re-oriented so that the two different devices form the rows and the expelled/non-expelled categories form the columns. There is no absolute rule about how such tables should be laid out, but in the author's experience, they are more intuitive if the independent factor is used as the columns and the dependent as the rows. This is what has been done above (expulsion may depend upon device design, but not vice versa). In some tables the two forms of categorization, though potentially associated, may not have any obvious dependent relationship and the table could equally well be presented in either orientation.

Table 16.1 A contingency table showing the effect of IUD design upon the number of women where the device was expelled

	Control design	Test design
Not expelled	1732 (86.6%)	1778 (88.9%)
Expelled	268 (13.4%)	222 (11.1%)

The percentage figures included in the table are column percentages. Thus, in the first column, 86.6 per cent of women using the control device did not expel the device and 13.4 per cent did. These indicate an apparently lower expulsion rate with the new test design.

16.1.2 The contingency chi-square test

The sample data may suggest that the new device is superior to the old one, but these are only samples and the apparent difference could have arisen as a result of random sampling error. We therefore need to set up and test a null hypothesis.

Our null hypothesis is that, in larger populations of users, the rates of expulsion would be identical. The test we will employ is the contingency chi-square test.

⎯◯ Contingency chi-square test

Compares two (or more) sets of observed proportions. Is there significant evidence of a difference?

16.1.3 What determines whether we obtain statistical significance?

Within this test, two aspects of the data will determine whether the evidence is adjudged significant:

1. *How strong is the contrast between the two outcomes?* If one sample indicated an expulsion rate only very marginally greater than the other, we would have to accept that such a small difference could be due to sampling error alone. However, a large difference would be difficult to explain away on this basis.

2. *How large are the samples?* If one device showed a 5 per cent expulsion rate and the other a rate of 10 per cent, but these percentages were based upon samples each containing only 20 individuals, then the actual number of expulsions detected would be 1 and 2. This would prove absolutely nothing – identical populations could easily yield such figures. However, if the rates of 5 and 10 per cent were based upon samples of 10 000 we would be comparing 500 vs 1000 expulsions – an entirely convincing contrast.

The test will produce a test statistic (χ^2), which will be converted into a P value. As with most tests, the stronger the evidence, the greater the test statistic and the lower the P value. Figure 16.1 summarizes the situation.

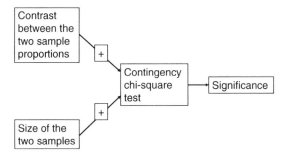

Figure 16.1   Factors influencing the outcome of a contingency chi-square test

16.1.4 Using a statistical package to perform the contingency chi-square test

Packages differ in the way in which they expect the data to be presented. Some will only accept the raw data. For our IUD trial, this would require a column with codes for the type of IUD each woman used (maybe 'C' or 'T' for control or test) and a second column with codes for the corresponding woman's outcome ('S' or 'F' for success/retained or 'F' for failed/expelled). There would then be 4000 rows of data – one for each subject.

Other packages will allow an alternative method where the data are entered in summarized format. In that case the data in Table 16.1 would simply occupy two rows of two columns. Notice however that only the actual counts should be used – not the percentages. If you are not clear just how important the last point is, just imagine entering the percentages. The analysis would have no indication whether the percentages were derived from 10 women given each treatment (nowhere near significant) or 10 million women (overwhelmingly significant).

⌐◯ Numbers *not* percentages

When entering data in summarized format, you must use the actual counts, not the percentages.

The next step will be to identify which columns contain the relevant data (either raw or summarized). Most packages produce pretty extensive output, but among it all should be the key results shown in Table 16.2.

The previous chapter mentioned the 'continuity' problem and introduced the Yates correction. Opinions are divided on the application of this correction to the contingency chi-square test. Some statistical packages offer both a corrected and an uncorrected result, others just the uncorrected. A commonly used stratagem is to quote the corrected result where the table contains only two columns and two rows,

Table 16.2 Generic output from a contingency chi-square analysis of rates of expulsion of two designs of IUD

Contingency chi-square test:	
Uncorrected chi-square = 4.921	$P = 0.027$
Corrected chi-square = 4.709	$P = 0.030$

but for larger tables to quote the uncorrected result. Fortunately, the correction makes very little difference unless we have results hovering on the verge of significance and the numbers involved are small. For large studies (such as the present case), the correction has only a very slight effect. Either way, the result is clearly significant.

The value of the test statistic (chi-square) may be included in a report of the outcome, but it is not vital.

16.2 Obtaining a 95 per cent CI for the change in the proportion of expulsions – is the difference large enough to be of practical significance?

Throughout this book, it has been emphasized that we should always try to go beyond statistical significance and also consider the extent of any difference and so assess practical significance. Unfortunately the chi-square test does not produce a 95 per cent CI for the extent of the difference. However, so long as we are only considering a 2×2 table, some packages (including Minitab) provide a separate routine to calculate a confidence interval.

If we are going to make any comments about practical significance, we should have established equivalence limits (in advance of seeing the results). It is known that rates of expulsion of IUDs may be influenced by all sorts of factors other than the design of the device. For example the precise positioning of the device in the uterus has a major influence. It had therefore been decided that any change in rates of expulsion would have to be at least 4 percentage points if it was to be considered as having real practical significance.

What you generally have to supply is the total numbers in each group (2000 in both cases with our example) and then you choose one category and quote the number in that category for both groups. In the example below, we will supply the numbers where expulsion did occur, i.e. 268 and 222, but supplying the numbers where it was retained would work just as well. You should then find that the confidence interval for the difference between the two rates of expulsions is 0.27–4.33 percentage points (see Figure 16.2). This confirms what the chi-square test had already discerned – a zero difference is excluded and so there is statistically significant evidence that the new design has performed better. However, the figure also shows that we cannot draw any absolutely definite conclusion as to the practical significance of the difference

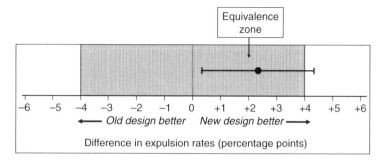

Figure 16.2   Difference in rates of expulsion of IUDs – almost certainly not of practical significance

between the two designs. The most optimistic view (extreme right-hand end of interval) is that the difference might just be great enough to be worthwhile, but realistically, the improvement achieved by this new design is very likely too small to be of real value.

⚷ 95 CI for the difference between two proportions

The chi-square test only assesses statistical significance. To assess practical significance, you will need a separate routine to calculate a 95 per cent CI for the difference between proportions.

16.3 Larger tables – attendance at diabetic clinics

In the example above there were only two groups to be compared (new and old design) and there were only two possible outcomes (IUD expelled or not expelled). The results could therefore be expressed in a contingency table with only two columns and two rows (a '2 × 2 table') This is the simplest experimental design and has much to recommend it, as the results are so easy to interpret. However, other experiments may be more complex. For example we might simultaneously compare more than two designs of IUD and/or there might be more than two outcomes (e.g. not expelled/expelled within 1 week/expelled after 1 week or more). The contingency chi-square test is easily extended to cover more complex designs.

As an example of a more complex case, we might want to compare various methods of encouraging diabetic patients to attend their next routine clinic appointment. During their May visit to the clinic, all patients will be issued with an appointment card that details when they should attend in June, but then various additional measures may be taken. Patients are randomly allocated to 4 groups:

Table 16.3 Attendance at a diabetes clinic following various additional reminders

	None	Verbal emphasis	Letter	Phone call
Attended	49 (65.3%)	53 (71.6%)	61 (83.6%)	65 (86.7%)
Did not attend	26 (34.7%)	21 (28.4%)	12 (16.4%)	10 (13.3%)

- no additional methods;

- verbal emphasis at end of May visit of the importance of attendance;

- letter in June;

- telephone call in June.

We then count those who do/do not attend their June appointment. The null hypothesis is that all four methods are equally effective. The results, expressed as a contingency table are shown in Table 16.3.

Ideally the total number allocated to each approach would have been the same. However, this was not quite achieved. This is not a problem, because the chi-square test takes account of different 'column totals'. For optimum power, extreme variation in group sizes should be avoided.

The column percentages have been included and visual inspection of these suggests that the rate of attendance is higher where additional reminders have been used, but a formal statistical test is required to see whether the differences within these small samples would continue to be seen in the longer term. The result of a contingency chi-square test will be a P value of 0.006 (highly significant).

16.3.1 The difficulty of interpreting the results from larger contingency tables

In the previous example, which produced results in a simple 2×2 table, the interpretation of the outcome was perfectly clear. However, in this case our results can no longer be summarized in a 2×2 table and the detailed interpretation of the outcome is problematic. We can reasonably conclude that at least one of the methods used is better than one of the others, but it is difficult to be any more specific. There are two extreme views that we might take:

- There are differences in effectiveness between all four methods of notification. Doing nothing is worst, a verbal emphasis is a bit better, a letter better still and a phone call best of all.

- There are only really two degrees of effect. Doing nothing and verbal emphasis are similarly ineffective and a letter or phone call produce about the same degree of improvement.

Various other views are also possible. The output from the contingency chi-square procedure is generally little help in choosing between interpretations. The moment we start doing experiments that go beyond the simple 2×2 contingency table design, our results become contentious and, the greater the degree of complexity, the less you will be able to conclude.

Sub-dividing large tables   Returning to our survey of possible reminders, let us assume that we propose to introduce a system of letters or phone calls, but are refused the necessary resources, so then it is verbal reminders or nothing. However, looking at Table 16.3, we suspect that, despite the statistical significance of the table as a whole, it is doubtful whether there is really any difference between doing nothing and the verbal reminders.

One (contentious) way to test such a question is to sub-divide the table. We could set up a simple 2×2 table consisting only of the data for 'none' and 'verbal emphasis'. A test of that reduced table gives $P = 0.409$. There is no evidence that verbal reminders would do any good. However, be careful with this approach. The sin of multiple-testing has already been condemned in Chapter 13, and Chapter 18 will emphasize the same refrain. If you start breaking down large contingency tables into smaller parts, any number could be created, leading to horrendous multiple testing. With the analysis suggested above, there was little risk of generating a false positive as we created only one sub-table. However, you definitely should not start with a large, non-significant table and break it up into numerous sub-tables and test them all with a view to finding something significant.

 Break a huge contingency table into every possible sub-table

You start with a massive table, but it emerges as non-significant. Break it up into every conceivable smaller table and test each one. Each sub-table may offer only a 5 per cent chance of a false positive, but with enough of them you are going to get lucky somewhere along the line.

Less experienced researchers gravitate to overly complex tables   In the author's experience, young, naive experimentalists commonly feel the need to perform hugely complex experiments with half a dozen different treatments and outcomes categorized into a similar number of possibilities. The results then form a 6×6 contingency table or something equally ridiculous. However hard one may try, these over-ambitious pioneers rarely accept warnings that their experimental results will be almost incapable of interpretation. They carry on blithely and it all ends in tears. There seems to be a sense that their research project would look pretty feeble if 3 months' work could be summarized in a measly 2 × 2 table – a bigger table would look much more impressive. Supervisors have a major role in constraining such misplaced ambition.

⚷ Keep it simple, keep it clear

Where possible, stick to simple experimental designs, where the results can be expressed as a 2 × 2 contingency table. The interpretation of the outcome will then be unambiguous.

16.4 Planning experimental size

16.4.1 Using a statistical package

For those commendably simple experiments that result in 2 × 2 contingency tables, some statistical packages include simple routines to calculate necessary sample size. For anything more complex, you are on your own – quite right too! The routine will require you to provide values for the following:

- the proportions anticipated in one of the groups to be considered;

- the difference between the two groups that should be detectable;

- The power required.

This is summarized in Figure 16.3. The first factor – proportion in group 1 – behaves in an unusual manner. Imagine the following cases. In each instance, we are trying to detect an increase in rates of success as we change from one treatment to another:

- change from 1 to 11 per cent;

- change from 45 to 55 per cent;

- change from 89 to 99 per cent.

In all cases, we are looking for the same 10 percentage points increase. It is reasonably obvious that the changes in the first and last scenarios should be pretty easy to pick out. In one case there is a 10-fold increase in successes and, in the latter, failures

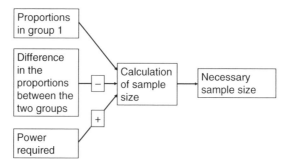

Figure 16.3 Calculation of necessary sample size for a contingency chi-square test

decrease 10-fold. Either of these changes will stand out prominently. However, in the intermediate situation, neither the successes nor the failures change dramatically. We would therefore require the greatest sample sizes where our proportions are around 50 per cent. This is therefore the one case where there is no simple positive or negative relationship between the factor and the outcome and no plus or minus label can be attached.

⊶ The middle ground is hardest

If we are starting with a very low proportion (near 0 per cent) or increasing to a very high proportion (near 100 per cent), the necessary sample size will be lowest.

If we are changing proportions, but staying around 50 per cent, the necessary sample size will be greatest.

The other two factors in Figure 16.3 behave in a more familiar manner. We know by now that small changes are hardest to detect, hence a negative. We also know that power is always positively associated with sample size – if you want more power you will need a larger sample size.

16.4.2 Calculating the necessary sample size for our IUD expulsion trial

To plan an appropriate size for the trial of two IUDs, we need to establish values for the following:

- *The proportion of expulsions in one of the groups* – literature reports suggest an expulsion rate of about 15 per cent for the control device.

- *The change that we would wish to detect* – we have already said that a change of four percentage points would be of practical significance. Therefore, if the new device reduced rates to 11 per cent, we would want to detect that change.

Table 16.4 Generic output from a calculation of necessary sample size for the IUD expulsion trial

Sample size for contingency chi-square test:	
Assumed P for group 1	0.15
Target P for group 2	0.11
Target power	0.95
Sample size (each group)	1835
Achieved power	0.95009

- *The required power* – let us go initially for the highest commonly used value (95 per cent) and, if that requires unachievable numbers, we will consider being a little less ambitious.

Generic output is then as in Table 16.4. The required sample size is 1835. Remember that this is for each treatment group, so we actually need a total of 3670 women. In the real world, we would need to start out with rather more, to allow for a proportion that cannot be followed up. Our original scheme was to use 2000 women in each group – so that was probably about right. As usual, no exact number of subjects delivers exactly the requested power and numbers are set to slightly over-achieve.

16.5 Chapter summary

A contingency table presents data that are based entirely upon categorization (both the columns and the rows are in this format). The contingency chi-square test is used to determine whether the proportion of individuals falling into a particular category changes according to the conditions. When performing this test the actual counts must be used. Where the data form a simple 2×2 table, the results of the test are unambiguously interpretable. The test can be applied to larger tables, but the interpretation will be less clear.

Many statistical packages provide a routine that will generate a 95 per cent CI for the extent of any change in a proportion within a 2×2 table and this can be used to check for practical significance. For experiments that can be described in a 2×2 contingency table, it is simple to calculate necessary sample sizes.

Part 4

Ordinal-scale data

17

Ordinal and non-normally distributed data. Transformations and non-parametric tests

> ### *This chapter will* ...
>
> - Describe the requirement for normally distributed data when using parametric tests (*t*-tests, ANOVAs and Pearson correlation)
>
> - Show how such tests can still be used and interpreted after data has been transformed to normality
>
> - Introduce non-parametric methods where data is converted to rankings, so they become 'distribution-free tests'
>
> - Explain why ordinal data is generally subjected to non-parametric tests
>
> - Discuss the appropriate wording of conclusions where a non-parametric test has proved significant
>
> - Describe how to decide whether data should be tested (i) directly, (ii) after transformation to normality or (iii) non-parametrically

Essential Statistics for the Pharmaceutical Sciences   Philip Rowe
© 2007 John Wiley & Sons, Ltd   ISBN 9780 470 03470 5 (HB)   ISBN 9780 470 03468 2 (PB)

- Describe four widely applicable non-parametric methods (Mann–Whitney, Wilcoxon paired samples, Krukal–Wallis and Spearman correlation)

In Chapter 5 we saw how the calculation of the 95 per cent CI for the mean can lead to nonsensical results if the data deviate severely from a normal distribution. This requirement for a normal distribution also applies to the *t*-tests, analyses of variance and correlation that we met in Chapters 6–14. These procedures are termed 'parametric methods' and are quite robust, so moderate non-normality does little damage, but in more extreme cases, some pretty dumb conclusions can emerge. This chapter looks at steps that can be taken to allow the analysis of seriously non-normal data and also of ordinal scale data.

17.1 Transforming data to a normal distribution

17.1.1 Production of a toxic metabolite in smokers and non-smokers

In a small minority of users, an analgesic produces a serious side-effect – inflammation of the liver. It is suspected that this may be due to a very minor, but toxic metabolite. It has been noted that the reaction is about twice as frequent among smokers compared with non-smokers. A theory is advanced that, because smoking induces greater levels of certain metabolic enzymes in the liver, the increased susceptibility among smokers might be due to the production of greater quantities of the toxic metabolite. If this theory were correct, then it ought to be possible to detect increased production of the rogue metabolite in smokers. Table 17.1 shows the amount of the relevant metabolite recovered in the urine of 20 smokers and non-smokers, following the ingestion of an oral dose (50 mg) of the drug. For now, focus on the first two columns and ignore the log data.

These quantities of metabolite are shown in Figure 17.1. There is a fairly strong visual impression that metabolite production is indeed higher among smokers, but unfortunately there is also a distinct impression that the data may not be normally distributed – there seems to be a scattering of high values above the main clusters of points. Figure 17.2 (a) provides an even stronger impression of positively skewed data with the smokers' data. Although not shown here, the non-smokers' data are similarly skewed.

If we were just to ignore this non-normality and perform a two-sample *t*-test on the raw data, the results would include a *P* value of 0.115, indicating a lack of statistical significance. However, we would be very unwise simply to accept this negative result, given that the test used is not appropriate for highly skewed data.

There are two possible solutions and we are going to look at both. The first is to use the same trick we saw in Chapter 5 – transformation.

Table 17.1 Production of a toxic metabolite (μg) from an analgesic drug in smokers and non-smokers

Smokers	Non-smokers	Log for smokers	Log for non-smokers
7.75	2.50	0.889	0.398
7.80	7.45	0.892	0.872
23.40	4.95	1.369	0.695
27.50	3.10	1.439	0.491
5.65	17.10	0.752	1.233
12.05	4.20	1.081	0.623
11.95	6.05	1.077	0.782
21.15	25.20	1.325	1.401
15.40	20.20	1.188	1.305
14.05	6.10	1.148	0.785
10.15	9.55	1.006	0.980
12.40	7.15	1.093	0.854
6.20	3.90	0.792	0.591
16.30	13.00	1.212	1.114
7.15	12.05	0.854	1.081
5.95	4.25	0.775	0.628
9.20	15.20	0.964	1.182
5.15	4.45	0.712	0.648
9.70	5.90	0.987	0.771
12.90	6.10	1.111	0.785

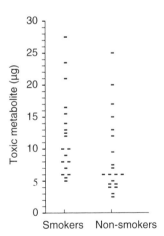

Figure 17.1 Production of a toxic metabolite from an analgesic drug in smokers and non-smokers

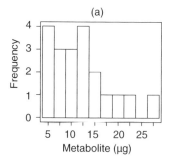 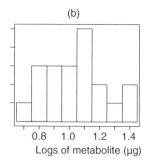

Figure 17.2 Histograms of (a) metabolite production and (b) logs of metabolite production from an analgesic drug in smokers

17.1.2 Carrying out a log transformation

We can try to find a mathematical transformation of the data that shows a better approximation to a normal distribution. With positive skew, either a square-root or a log transform may be useful. With this data, the square-root transform is insufficiently powerful and the data remain distinctly skewed. The results of the more powerful log transform are presented in Table 17.1 and Figure 17.2(b). The latter shows that the distribution for the smokers' data is now much more symmetrical. The effect on the non-smokers' data is not shown but is also satisfactory. We would then perform a standard two sample t-test, but apply it to the last two columns in Table 17.1. Generic output is shown in Table 17.2.

Wonder of wonders! Data that were non-significant are now revealed as significant ($P = 0.034$). It is usually at about this point that the cynical cry 'cheat!' How dare we use this statistical fiddle to convert non-significant results into significant ones? Essentially, we need have no qualms about this approach. It is entirely respectable and is definitely superior to the analysis of the original data, because the transformed data are much closer to a normal distribution. The only caveat would be that, if we are

Table 17.2 Generic output for a two-sample t-test comparing the logs of the amounts of toxic metabolite produced by smokers and non-smokers (last two columns of Table 17.1)

Two-sample t-test	
Mean (log smoke)	1.033
Mean (log non-smoke)	0.861
Difference (log smoke – log non-smoke)	0.172
95 per cent CI difference	0.014–0.331
P	0.034

going to do this kind of thing, we should ideally declare our intentions in advance. It is not good practice to gather data and then thrash around trying every possible statistical approach until we find one that produces the desired result (generally a significant one!).

⚷ Carrying out tests on transformed data

It is normal and legitimate practice to use transformations to convert data to a better approximation of a normal distribution and then carry out tests on the transformed data.

The contrast between the successful outcome when testing the normally distributed transformed data and the failure with the highly skewed raw data is an example of the large loss of power that often accompanies the application of procedures such as a *t*-test to inappropriate data.

⚷ Major loss of power with inappropriate data

It is quite common to suffer a large loss of power if highly skewed or otherwise non-normal data are analysed by methods that assume normality.

If we want to comment upon the size of the difference between smokers and non-smokers, we need to be very careful in interpreting these results. The limits of the 95 per cent CI for the difference between the two groups are reported as 0.0140–0.3307. However, these were calculated from log-transformed data and need to be converted back to their antilogs. This then gives a CI of 1.03–2.14. However, these differences were arrived at by subtracting one log value from another and then taking the anti-log. When you carry out that procedure, you are actually performing a division. Consequently, the numbers we end up with are not the differences in numbers of micrograms of toxin produced, they are the ratios between toxin production in the two groups. The correct interpretation is that we can be 95 per cent confident that the smokers produce between 1.03 and 2.14 times more toxin than the non-smokers. In such a case, the null hypothesis should be expressed as 'The ratio of toxin production in smokers to that in non-smokers is 1.0'. Statistical significance is then based on the fact that the 95 per cent CI does not include the figure of 1.0.

The point estimate for the effect size is subject to the same logic. The estimated difference is given as 0.172 and the antilog of that is 1.49. Therefore, it is estimated that smokers produce about 50 per cent more toxin. The point estimate and 95 per cent CI for the effect of smoking are shown in Figure 17.3.

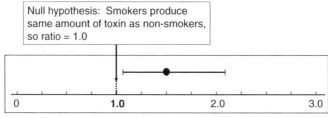

Ratio of toxin production in smokers to non-smokers

Figure 17.3   The 95 per cent confidence interval for the ratio between toxin production in smokers and non-smokers

---

Effect size when a log transform has been used

We obtain a 95 per cent CI for the ratio between the two means, rather than their absolute difference.

17.2 The Mann–Whitney test – a non-parametric method

17.2.1   A substitute for the two-sample *t*-Test

Instead of transforming the data to normality, we could employ one of a range of procedures referred to as 'non-parametric tests'. These partially duplicate the functionality of tests we have already met, but use a method of calculation that does not depend upon a normal distribution. The non-parametric test that is generally substituted for the two sample *t*-test goes by a variety of names, but is most commonly called the 'Mann–Whitney' test.

17.2.2   Converting data to rankings

The defining characteristic of all non-parametric tests is that we take the data and convert it into ranks. To convert the toxin data we start with the actual quantities of toxin produced (forget about the log-transformed data for this test), and search through it looking for the lowest single value. This turns out to be the value of 2.5 µg for the first of the non-smokers, so this is awarded the rank value of 1. The next lowest values (3.10, 3.90, 4.20, 4.25, 4.45 and 4.95) are also among non-smokers and get ranks of 2, 3, 4, 5, 6 and 7. The next value is then for one of the smokers (5.15) and it gets rank 8. This process continues simply enough for the lowest 12 values, but then we find that the next value (6.10) occurs twice (among

Table 17.3 Conversion of quantities of toxin into rank values

Smokers		Non-smokers	
Toxin (μg)	Rank	Toxin (μg)	Rank
7.75	19	2.50	1
7.80	20	7.45	18
23.40	38	4.95	7
27.50	40	3.10	2
5.65	9	17.10	35
12.05	26.5	4.20	4
11.95	25	6.05	12
21.15	37	25.20	39
15.40	33	20.20	36
14.05	31	6.10	13.5
10.15	24	9.55	22
12.40	28	7.15	16.5
6.20	15	3.90	3
16.30	34	13.00	30
7.15	16.5	12.05	26.5
5.95	11	4.25	5
9.20	21	15.20	32
5.15	8	4.45	6
9.70	23	5.90	10
12.90	29	6.10	13.5
Rank total	488		332

the non-smokers). These are referred to as tied values. They should get ranks 13 and 14, but there is no logical reason why one should be ranked higher than the other, so they each receive a rank of 13.5. We eventually reach the highest value (27.5), which is for one of the smokers, and it gets rank 40. The original data and their rankings are shown in Table 17.3.

☞ Non-parametric tests are based upon ranks

In non-parametric tests the data are transformed into rank values and then all further calculations are based solely upon these rankings.

17.2.3 Using rankings for further calculation

All further calculations are then carried out on these rank values rather than on the original data. The next stage is to add up all the rank values for the two groups to produce 'rank totals'. On a null hypothesis that there is no systematic difference between smokers and non-smokers, we would expect high and low rank values to be scattered randomly between the two groups and the rank totals to be fairly similar. However, if (as we suspect) the higher values are generally among the smokers, then this is where we will also find the highest rank values and the higher rank total. The rank totals shown above (488 and 332) hint fairly strongly at a difference, but is the difference big enough to be convincing? The rest of the Mann–Whitney test answers precisely that question.

17.2.4 Conducting a Mann–Whitney test

Depending upon the particular statistical package used, the data may be entered either in two columns or all in a single column with a separate column containing codes indicating which groups the values belong to. What you enter are the actual quantities of toxin produced; you do not have to work out the rankings – that should all be done by the statistical package.

Output (Table 17.4) varies from package to package, but generally includes a median value for each group. Note that, while these are useful descriptively, they do not enter into the calculation of the test. There are likely to be two P values. This arises because there were some tied values among the data. The existence of ties somewhat undermines the method of calculation used within the Mann–Whitney test and it is possible to apply a correction to compensate for this. The general preference seems to be for the latter value (labelled as 'adjusted for ties'), but unless there are a huge number of ties the difference is not usually great. In this case there are so few ties (three pairs) that the two P values are apparently identical and the result is significant either way.

17.2.5 Interpreting a significant outcome

When a t-test produces a significant outcome, its interpretation is quite straightforward – there is evidence that the two population mean values differ. Unfortunately, with non-parametric tests such as Mann–Whitney, it is not so simple. The conclusion

Table 17.4 Generic output from a Mann–Whitney test of the amounts of toxin produced by smokers and non-smokers

Mann–Whitney:	
Median (smoke)	11.05
Median (non-smoke)	6.10
P	0.036
P (adjusted for ties)	0.036

may be worded simply in terms of evidence of an increase/decrease in values, or we may want to be more specific and talk about changes in the median or mean.

Strictly speaking, because no mean or median is even calculated as part of the test, the null hypothesis should be that:

'Smokers and non-smokers produce the same amounts of toxic metabolite.'

What this is understood to mean is that, if we randomly selected one smoker and one non-smoker, the chances that the smoker would produce more toxin than the non-smoker is exactly equal to the chances of the opposite pattern. That way we make no reference to the mean, median or any other statistical parameter.

As the null hypothesis has been dismissed, we have evidence that there must be a difference in the amount of toxin produced. Based on Figure 17.1, we can conclude that:

'Smokers tend to produce more toxin than non-smokers.'

That would be a minimum conclusion that nobody is likely to challenge. Can we then go on and say that this must also imply an increase in the median or mean amount produced?

- *The median* – in the majority of cases a demonstration of generally increased (or decreased) values can be taken to imply a corresponding change in the median. However, just be aware that there are some bizarre distributions (usually involving extreme skewness) where the median may not change in the way you would anticipate (see Appendix 1 to this chapter)

- *The mean* – the process of ranking destroys all information regarding the absolute magnitude of the individual results and consequently it would be very risky to try to claim that a Mann–Whitney test had demonstrated a change in the mean. To justify such a conclusion, you would have to make such extensive assumptions about the distribution of the data that you could probably use a parametric test anyway!

➔⊙ Interpreting a significant Mann–Whitney test

'*Values are generally higher in this group than in that*'– this makes no assumptions about how the data is distributed. Minimum claim – little risk.

'*The median is greater in this group than in that*' – only assumption is that the data is not distributed in a totally bizarre manner. Generally OK, but check with an expert if the data sets have extreme distributions.

'*The mean is greater in this group than in that*'– rarely justifiable.

17.2.6   Choosing – parametric or non-parametric?

When non-parametric methods are applied to data that is normally distributed, they are slightly less powerful than their parametric equivalents, although the difference is not great. For the tests covered in this chapter, the non-parametric test has about 95 per cent of the power of its parametric equivalent. In other words, if our data is normally distributed then a sample of 19 tested by a parametric method would provide about the same power as a sample of 20 tested by the non-parametric equivalent. Since the power of the two types of test is so similar, it is not surprising that the P values generated [0.034 for the t-test (when applied to the transformed data) and 0.036 for the Mann–Whitney test] are barely different.

However, if the data is severely non-normal we can lose a huge amount of power by using a parametric test. We saw this loss of power when we obtained a non-significant result by applying a t-test to the untransformed (and highly skewed) toxin data.

⚷ Strengths of parametric and non-parametric tests

Parametric – slightly more powerful than non-parametric where data is reasonably normally distributed and they produce a 95 per cent CI for the size of the experimental effect.
Non-parametric – may be much more powerful than parametric tests if data is seriously non-normal.

A good general rule is to use a parametric test whenever possible even if that necessitates a transformation of the data. However, some data sets are such a mess that no amount of jiggery-pokery will render them normal and in these cases a non-parametric test is our ultimate fall-back.

⚷ Dealing with non-normally distributed data

First choice – convert to normal distribution by transformation and use a parametric test.
Second choice – resort to a non-parametric test.

17.2.7   'Distribution-free tests'

When we convert measurement data to rankings, we destroy all information about the distribution of the data. For instance, when we ranked the toxin measurements, all that remained was a series of ranks from 1 to 40 and we would have got exactly the same set of values regardless of whether the original distribution was normal, skewed, bimodal or any other shape. Because ranked data are blind to the initial distribution, the non-parametric tests are sometimes called 'distribution-free tests'.

17.3 Dealing with ordinal data

Back in Chapter 1, data were described as 'interval' (measurements on a regular scale), 'ordinal' (measurements on a scale of undefined steps) and 'nominal' (classifications). We have dealt extensively with two of these, but ordinal data have thus far been ignored.

17.3.1 Why ordinal data are generally analysed by non-parametric methods

Ordinal data typically include things like patients' subjective descriptions of their condition. A score may be allocated, ranging from 1 to 4, where:

1 = no/almost no pain
2 = slight pain
3 = significant pain
4 = severe pain

Ordinal data tend not to form normal distributions. For a start, it is often recorded on scales with a very limited number of possible values. Scales of four, five or six points are frequently seen. In such cases, it is impossible for the data to form the sort of smooth, bell-shaped distribution that constitutes a true normal distribution. However, then the problem is further exacerbated. Although there is no necessary reason for it, anybody who has worked with real-world, ordinal data knows that it is frequently hideously non-normal. Offered a scale of possible scores, people will quite frequently do bizarre things like only using the extreme upper and lower values but not the middle ones, or else they will produce a completely flat distribution, with no peak frequencies anywhere. No amount of mathematical transformation is going to convert that sort of mess into anything remotely resembling a normal distribution.

⚏⊙ It is normal to be non-normal

It is theoretically possible for ordinal scale data to approximate a normal distribution, but marked non-normality is all too common.

There is no absolute case that parametric methods cannot be used with ordinal scale data. If the scoring system allows a reasonably wide range of possible values and if these happen to approximate a normal distribution, parametric methods could be used. However the reality of working with ordinal data is:

- frequently horribly non-normal distributions;

- a small potential gain in power if a parametric method is deployed with data that are reasonably normal;

- a very large potential loss of power if a parametric method is used with data that are badly non-normal.

A common view is that, when planning any experiment where data will be collected on an ordinal scale, we may as well reconcile ourselves to the use of non-parametric methods from the outset.

⊶⊙ Dealing with ordinal scale data

Unless there is specific evidence that the data is likely to behave itself unusually well, just accept that non-parametric methods will have to be used. Power loss will, at worst, be very slight.

17.3.2 An example of dealing with ordinal scale data – applying the Mann–Whitney test to the effectiveness of an analgesic

Two teams of volunteers rate the effectiveness of either an active herbal analgesic or a placebo for the treatment of mild pain. The design is unpaired – one team are allocated to active and the other to placebo tablets. The scale used to report effectiveness is:

4 = completely/Almost completely effective
3 = strongly effective
2 = moderately effective
1 = slightly effective
0 = no/almost no effect

The results are shown in Table 17.5 and graphically in Figure 17.4. Two things are apparent:

1. There is a strong impression that the active preparation is receiving higher scores than the placebo, but formal testing is still required.

Table 17.5 Scores for effectiveness of placebo/active analgesic

Placebo	Active
3, 0, 2, 4, 0	1, 3, 3, 3, 4,
0, 2, 0, 0, 1,	4, 3, 0, 4, 3,
1, 0, 0, 0, 3,	4, 4, 3, 1, 2,
2, 1, 2, 1, 3	4, 4, 3, 2, 2

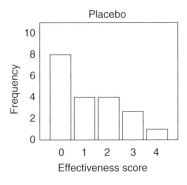 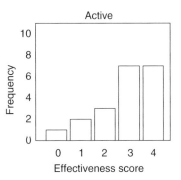

Figure 17.4 Effectiveness of placebo or active analgesic

2. Both distributions are strongly skewed, but as one shows positive and the other negative skew, there is no way we are going to be able to transform them both to normality.

17.3.3 Analysing the results

With an unpaired design and measurements on an interval scale, we would have used a two-sample *t*-test to check for any difference. However, this data are ordinal and not remotely normally distributed, so we will have to move to its non-parametric equivalent – the Mann–Whitney test.

The result of a Man–Whitney test on this data is an uncorrected *P* value of 0.0008. There are many tied values in this set of results and adjusting for ties does now slightly reduce *P* to 0.0006. Either way the result is strongly significant.

As explained previously, the significant result can certainly be interpreted as evidence that the active preparation generally had a greater effect than the placebo and a more detailed claim that the active preparation had a greater median effect is pretty uncontroversial, even with these rather skew distributions.

17.4 Other non-parametric methods

There are huge numbers of other non-parametric tests available. Three are especially useful as substitutes for parametric tests that have already been covered in this book.

Table 17.6 Haemoglobin levels (g/l) in a group of vegans before and after vitamin B12 supplementation

Pre-treatment	Post-treatment	Change
142	146	+4
140	160	+20
135	143	+8
153	153	0
136	155	+19
142	141	−1
146	151	+5
117	133	+16
139	139	0
156	153	−3
154	155	+1
152	150	−2
154	156	+2
133	155	+22
146	151	+5
153	153	0
126	140	+14
115	114	−1
159	164	+5
146	152	+6
136	142	+6
158	161	+3
129	144	+15
137	152	+15
150	153	+3
136	141	+5
137	149	+12
136	151	+15

17.4.1 Wilcoxon paired samples test – a substitute for the paired *t*-test

In the paired *t*-test we calculate the change in a measured end-point for each individual and the test expects these differences to form a normal distribution. If this condition is not met, the Wilcoxon paired samples test can be used instead.

As an example, we will consider (Table 17.6) some changes that occurred in haemoglobin levels in a group of vegans when given vitamin B12 supplementation. The study was paired, each individual providing a pre-treatment blood sample and then a further sample after 4 weeks of supplementation.

Figure 17.5 shows this to be a very difficult data set, with a strong suspicion of a bimodal distribution. Such a distribution is biologically quite credible – there may well be a majority whose diet already contains adequate B12 in whom supplementation

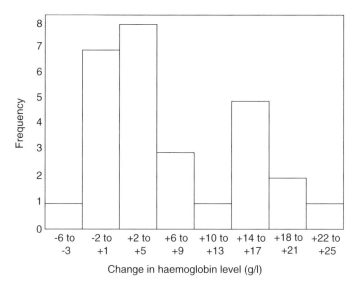

Figure 17.5 Histogram of changes in haemoglobin levels after vitamin B12 treatment

will be associated with small random changes clustered around zero, but a minority (approximately 30 per cent) who are deficient and where we see decisive increases in haemoglobin levels.

Figure 17.5 strongly suggests that this treatment is much more likely to lead to an increase than to a decrease in haemoglobin levels, but a formal test is required. No transformation is going to convert this to a normal distribution. With normally distributed changes, we would have used a paired *t*-test, but with this data we will change to the Wilcoxon paired sample test.

The test is directly available in some statistical packages (e.g. SPSS) but not in others such as Minitab. Where it is available, the pre- and post-treatment values are entered into two columns and the test can be performed directly. With the likes of Minitab, the test can be achieved, but it is messy. You will first have to calculate the change that occurs in each individual and enter these into a column. Then the 'one-sample Wilcoxon' procedure is used to compare these values against a null hypothesis of no systematic change.

The output obtained varies so much between packages that there is no such thing as generic output. However, among whatever you do get, there should be a *P* value of <0.001. There is significant evidence that B12 has an effect on haemoglobin values.

17.4.2 Kruskal–Wallis test – a substitute for the one-way ANOVA

This acts as an equivalent of the one-way ANOVA that we met in Chapter 13. The requirements underlying the ANOVA are that all the populations from which

Table 17.7   Pain scores with three different analgesics

Oxycodone	Morphine	Diamorphine
64	62	23
71	50	42
21	76	30
75	51	70
12	45	71
11	35	65
15	54	35
20	71	20
69	31	25
38	49	45
9	19	9
10	10	15
74	55	47
79	80	6
17	15	15
32	62	14
15	31	15
51	80	17
72	41	20
64	19	25

samples are drawn should be normally distributed and have equal SDs. The Kruskal–Wallis test allows us to circumvent these requirements.

To illustrate the test, consider a trial of analgesia in palliative care. Sixty patients are randomized into three groups. One group receives oxycodone, one morphine and the final group diamorphine. Over the next 5 days, the dosage is adjusted to what is considered the optimum for each patient. The patients then score their pain on a 'visual analogue' scale. This consists of a line on a piece of paper. One end of the line is labelled 'no pain' and the other 'severe pain'. The patient then makes a pencil mark on the line at a point indicating their impression of their pain. The scale is 10 cm long and the distance is measured to the nearest mm, giving potential scores from zero to 100. The results are shown in Table 17.7.

The data are ordinal and, with only 20 observations for each drug, a histogram would provide little guidance as to whether the data are normally distributed. Under these circumstances, it would be risky to assume a normal distribution. The non-parametric Kruskal–Wallis test is preferable to a one-way analysis of variance.

To perform this test, most statistical packages require all the data to be entered into a single column with a further column contains codes indicating which group a result belongs to (as described for the one-way ANOVA). Generic output is shown in Table 17.8.

Table 17.8 Generic output from a Kruskal–Wallis test of pain scores with different analgesics

Kruskal–Wallis: Analgesic	Median pain score
Oxycodone	35.0
Morphine	49.5
Diamorphine	24.0
$P = 0.097$	
P (adjusted for ties) $= 0.097$	

The median pain scores suggest a considerable difference between these drugs. However, the apparent contrasts are not statistically significant.

With the one-way ANOVA, most statistical packages implement a series of follow-up tests to determine exactly where any differences lie. Similar procedures exist to allow follow-up after a significant Kruskal–Wallis test, but unfortunately they are not widely implemented in statistical packages. There would be no point in doing so in the present case, but if another data set proves significant and you want to perform follow-up tests, you will either have to resort to a very powerful (and probably not very friendly) statistical package, or do the calculation manually. The latter is tedious, but recipes are available. (A clear account is available in Zar J.H., 1999, *Biostatistical Analysis*, Prentice Hall, NJ; pp. 223–226.)

17.4.3 Spearman correlation – a substitute for Pearson correlation

Technically, Pearson correlation (Chapter 14) does have an assumption that the two sets of data are normally distributed, but it is pretty rare to see anybody bothering to check whether they actually are and there is precious little evidence of anything going radically wrong if they are not. However, non-parametric Spearman correlation is quite frequently resorted to with ordinal data.

To illustrate its use we will look at an investigation of a new explanatory leaflet. A previous version of the leaflet proved difficult to understand for patients with restricted educational achievement. The new version was drawn up by a specialist consultant (at great expense) and is supposed to be generally clearer and, crucially, equally accessible to all users. To test it, patients with a wide spectrum of educational achievement are asked to read the new leaflet and then answer five knowledge-testing questions. Each patient is then awarded a knowledge score of between 0 and 5. The patients are also allocated an education score of between 1 and 6 (1 for those with no formal educational qualifications; 6 for graduates with additional professional qualifications). The education and knowledge scores, along with their rankings, are shown in Table 17.9.

Table 17.9 Educational levels and knowledge scores after reading
revised information leaflet

Education Score	Knowledge score	Ranked education score	Ranked knowledge score
1	0	2.0	1.0
1	3	2.0	8.0
1	1	2.0	3.0
2	3	4.5	8.0
2	1	4.5	3.0
3	1	7.5	3.0
3	3	7.5	8.0
3	4	7.5	12.0
3	3	7.5	8.0
4	4	11.0	12.0
4	5	11.0	16.0
4	3	11.0	8.0
5	5	14.5	16.0
5	5	14.5	16.0
5	2	14.5	5.0
5	4	14.5	12.0
6	5	17.5	16.0
6	5	17.5	16.0

Figure 17.5 suggests that we are still not doing a very good job – there are an awful lot of low scores. We also appear to have failed to achieve equal accessibility – there is a strong suspicion that those with lower educational levels are also achieving poorer knowledge scores.

To test for a relationship between educational level and amount gleaned from the leaflet, we need some from of correlation analysis. Both characteristics are assessed on ordinal scales with a very limited range of possible values, so we would probably use non-parametric Spearman correlation.

The procedure is directly implemented in SPSS, but not in Minitab. In the latter case, it can still be performed, but it is a bit of a cludge. With packages where the test is directly available, the data are simply entered into two columns and the appropriate test selected. With other packages, we proceed in two stages – first convert the education and knowledge scores into rankings and then perform Pearson correlation on the rankings. As rankings are being used, the overall procedure will constitute Spearman correlation.

Convert the data to ranks Your statistical package may contain a routine to automate the process of calculating rankings from your data, otherwise it will have to be done manually. (Minitab can be used to do this – in the menu structure, go to

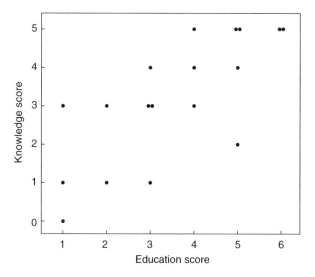

Figure 17.6 Relationship between educational level and score for knowledge after reading information leaflet

'Data' and then 'Rank'.) To perform ranking manually see Section 17.2.2. Table 17.9 includes the rankings.

Carry out correlation analysis of the ranking values   Correlation is carried out in the usual way, indicating the two columns containing the rankings. Results will be as in Table 17.10. If you are using a package that offers Spearman correlation, the fact that it is Spearman correlation will probably be indicated. Unfortunately, with a package like Minitab, where we needed a work-around, the program will not be aware that the data you fed it were actually a series of rankings, so the output may say 'Pearson correlation' when this is now in fact Spearman correlation.

The Spearman correlation coefficient works in essentially the same way as Pearson's. Its value can be anything between -1 and $+1$. Zero represents no correlation and the extreme values either perfect negative or perfect positive correlation. In this case, a Spearman correlation coefficient of $+0.748$ indicates quite a strong relationship. The P value is strongly significant, so it looks as if we were wasting our money when we hired the consultant (how unusual is that?).

Table 17.10   Generic output for Spearman correlation analysis of education scores and knowledge scores

Spearman correlation:

Correlation of education and knowledge $= +0.748$
$P < 0.001$

🔑 Non-parametric equivalents of other procedures

Parametric	*Non-parametric*
Two-sample *t*-test:	Mann–Whitney test
Paired *t*-test:	Wilcoxon paired samples test
One-way ANOVA:	Kruskal–Wallis test
Pearson correlation:	Spearman correlation

17.5 Chapter summary

t-Tests, analyses of variance and Pearson correlation are referred to as 'parametric methods' and they all make an assumption that data will be normally distributed. These (especially the first two) can be very misleading if applied to severely non-normal data.

Data may be converted to a normal distribution using log transforms, etc., as described in Chapter 5. Strongly positively skewed data are often converted to a normal distribution by log transformation. When this is done to allow analysis by a two-sample *t*-test, you should be aware that the 95 per cent CI for the size of the treatment effect will estimate the ratio between the values of the endpoint under the two conditions instead of the absolute difference in the value.

An alternative approach is to use a non-parametric test that does the same job as one of the parametric tests. These tests convert the data to rankings and the distribution of the data (largely) ceases to be an issue. They are sometimes called 'distribution-free tests'.

A significant result from a non-parametric equivalent of a *t*-test or an analysis of variance can always be interpreted as evidence of a change in values. Beyond that, so long as the data are not very awkwardly distributed (e.g. extremely skew), a significant result can be interpreted as evidence of a change in the median.

Where data are reasonably normally distributed, non-parametric methods are a little less powerful than their parametric equivalents, but where the data are severely non-normal, the non-parametric test may be much more powerful. With non-normally distributed interval scale data, the best solution is transformation to normality, but failing that, non-parametric methods can be used with only modest loss of power.

Ordinal data can potentially approximate to a normal distribution, but tends to be severely non-normal. The use of non-parametric methods is not obligatory with such data, but is common practice.

Four non-parametric tests are briefly introduced:

1. Mann–Whitney test equivalent to the two-sample *t*-test;

2. Wilcoxon paired samples test equivalent to the paired *t*-test;

3. Kruskal–Wallis test equivalent to the one-way ANOVA;

4. Spearman correlation equivalent to Pearson correlation.

Appendix to chapter 17

Do not assume that a significant result from a non-parametric test can necessarily be interpreted as evidence of a difference in median values.

Despite what some books claim, it is *not* safe to assume that a significant Mann–Whitney test can always be interpreted as evidence of a difference in the medians for the two groups being compared. Table 17.11 shows self-assessed severity scores for gastro-intestinal discomfort in groups of 50 patients taking two different analgesic drugs. The scoring is:

0 = none/virtually none;
1 = mild;
2 = moderate;
3 = severe.

The data are ordinal and extremely positively skewed, with a majority of zero scores and a tail of other scores on one side only. Group 2 appears to have somewhat higher scores (22 positive scores compared with only 11 in group 1). For a formal comparison, we would use the non-parametric Mann–Whitney test. That yields a *P* value (adjusted for ties) of 0.021, so there is significant evidence of higher scores in group 2.

More than half of each group has a score of zero, so the median score must perforce be zero in both cases. So, while it is OK to conclude that 'scores are higher in group 2 than group 1', you certainly could not claim that 'group 2 has a higher median score' – the median is zero for both groups.

Table 17.11 Gastro-intestinal discomfort scores in patients taking two different analgesic drugs

Discomfort score	Number reporting this score (drug 1)	(drug 2)
0	39	28
1	6	12
2	4	6
3	1	4

Part 5

Some challenges from the real world

18
Multiple testing

This chapter will . . .

- Explain what multiple testing is and why it is a problem

- Describe the circumstances in which it is most likely to arise

- Review methods that can be used to prevent false conclusions being relied upon

---

18.1 What is it and why is it a problem?

With every statistical test we perform, we face the fact that if no real effect were present, there would still be a 5 per cent risk of a false positive. We accept this small risk along with every *t*-test or correlation analysis, etc. The real problem comes when we indulge in a plethora of tests and the generic term 'multiple testing' covers this scenario. It is one thing learning to live with the standard 5 per cent risk, but multiple tests will jointly entail a much greater hazard that, somewhere, a false positive will creep in.

Taken to extremes, multiple testing is virtually guaranteed to find 'statistical significance' even in the absence of any real effects. For example, we could measure 10 different endpoints in a series of people (height, blood pressure, hand-grip strength, etc.) and those endpoints might be entirely independent of one another. We could then test for significant correlation between all possible pairs of endpoints.

Essential Statistics for the Pharmaceutical Sciences Philip Rowe
© 2007 John Wiley & Sons, Ltd   ISBN 9780470 03470 5 (HB)   ISBN 9780 470 03468 2 (PB)

This would require 45 analyses, each carrying the standard 5 per cent risk. The chances of hitting at least one meaningless (but apparently significant) correlation would then be about 90 per cent.

In most cases multiple testing arises from naivety, but in others it is the product of overzealous searching for statistical significance and no doubt there is a hardcore of outright villainy – the sure and certain knowledge that if you do enough tests, you are bound to get lucky eventually.

⚷ Multiple testing

A single statistical test carries a 5 per cent risk of producing a false positive conclusion – generally considered an acceptable level of risk.

Repeated tests rack up a much greater (and ultimately unacceptable) risk.

In this chapter, we will first review the situations where multiple testing can arise and then look at various stratagems that should help avoid excessive risks of false positives.

18.2 Where does multiple testing arise?

The commoner sources of this problem are:

- comparing several treatments against each other;

- recording numerous endpoints and testing each one for changes;

- measuring the same end point on several occasions and testing at each time point;

- breaking the data into numerous sub-sets and testing within each of these.

We will look briefly at each of these.

18.2.1 Comparing several treatments

Within a single piece of work, we might assess several possible treatments and measure the same endpoint for each treatment. If the endpoint is a measured variable, a t-test for each possible pair of treatments might look tempting or, with a categorical endpoint, repeated chi-square tests. The potential for multiple testing rises rapidly if we insist on making every possible comparison among three, four, five, etc. different treatments.

18.2.2 Comparing several endpoints

Even when comparing just two treatments, there may be a whole raft of endpoints. When comparing two chemical products, we might measure the levels of large numbers of impurities. Similarly in a biological setting, we might want to see whether a dietary change alters blood lipids and end up measuring triglycerides, total cholesterol and high, low and very low density lipoprotein cholesterol. If we performed separate t-tests on each impurity or each type of lipid, we would run a considerable risk of detecting false differences.

18.2.3 Testing at several time points

Particularly in biological and medical experiments, we frequently determine the relevant endpoint at several time points. Therefore, we might take a group who begin yoga and a control group who do not, and measure subjects' blood pressure every month for the following year. If we then carried out t-tests (control vs yoga) at each of the 12 monthly observation points, we would again run an elevated risk of false positives.

18.2.4 Testing within numerous sub-groups

This is one of the worst danger areas for multiple testing. Problems arise if we experiment on a mixed bag of subjects and then start breaking the subjects down into sub-groups based on their gender, age, ethnicity, disease status or whatever. When testing a medical treatment, we might start with a single statistical analysis based on the whole data set, which is perfectly respectable. If that fails to achieve significance, we might then think 'Well, maybe this stuff only works in people of a certain age', so we divide the data into six subsets each containing subjects in the same decade of life. We then compare controls vs actively treated within each age group separately. We now have a significant degree of multiplicity and are likely to 'discover' that (say) subjects aged 60–69 are responsive to our treatment, even if nobody else is. If that does not work then we could subdivide by gender (two sub-groups) or the severity of disease (mild, moderate, severe – three sub-groups). The real killer is to start combining several criteria. In the case above we could potentially generate $6 \times 2 \times 3 = 36$ sub-groups ranging from males, aged 20–29 with mild disease to females, aged 70–79 with severe disease. With 36 sub-groups, it would be very surprising if none of them generated an apparently significant effect.

   If an honest author describes the analysis of half a dozen different end-points or 20 sub-group analyses, one of which is significant, then the multiplicity is overt and an educated reader can be suitably cautious. However, the unscrupulous may conduct endless analyses and only report the one that hit the jackpot – covert multiplicity. The latter is out-and-out dishonesty – you might as well just make the results up! Against covert multiple testing, the reader will remain pretty much defenceless until journals upgrade their procedures (see Section 18.4).

 Break the data down into large numbers of sub-groups and publish the one that produces a 'significant' result

Wicked! The effectiveness of this one depends only on how unscrupulous you are prepared to be. If you are prepared simply to publish the sub-group that best suits your purposes and keep quiet about the fact that it was part of a larger experiment, there is no limit to what you can prove. Those with some residual scruples may prefer to own up to the full data set, but invent some spurious reason why there is justification for focusing on the particular sub-group where a significant result was obtained.

   This trick works best where there are plenty of apparently logical reasons for sub-dividing the data and human data is ideal for this. Subdivide by gender, age, ethnicity, social class and disease status (or any combination of these) and when you find that your new treatment reduces blood pressure to a statistically significant extent among Caucasian, Protestant, males aged 35–55 who also suffer from migraine, then this is obviously the group upon whom we should especially focus.

18.3 Methods to avoid false positives

18.3.1 Use a single ('omnibus') test to avoid a series of pair-wise comparisons

Multiple treatments   Where we have compared several different treatments, record-ing the same endpoint for each one, an omnibus test should generally be the first step in analysis. If an experiment addresses the question of whether a measured variable changes under a range of different conditions, we have already seen (Chapter 13) that a single analysis of variance will avoid the problems that would arise with repeated *t*-tests. If the omnibus test proves significant, then we can start digging into the detail to find out which treatment differs from which other. We have seen that a Dunnett's or Tukey's test can legitimately be used to make detailed comparisons.

Multiple endpoints   For this scenario, there is a whole other area of analysis referred to as 'multivariate' statistics. These methods also allow omnibus testing – all end-points are considered simultaneously. Multivariate stats are among the most com-plex to perform and interpret – there are generally six different ways to do any one job! However, do not be put off. Multivariate stats can uncover subtle effects that you would never find by looking at each endpoint in isolation. What you will need is seriously competent statistical advice.

Multiple time points   With observations at several time points, all the data can be considered simultaneously using a technique called repeated measures analysis of variance. This can be carried out using Minitab. Its execution and interpretation is not unduly complex, but is probably best undertaken with expert statistical support.

18.3.2 The Bonferroni correction

Bonferroni keeps the rate of type I errors down to 5 per cent...   In many instances, omnibus tests are not possible. If there are several comparisons to be made, each involving different groups of individuals and different endpoints, there may be no choice but to use a series of discrete statistical tests. In these circumstances, the Bonferroni correction may be applied to maintain the overall risk of false positives at the standard level of 5 per cent.

What the Bonferroni correction does is to raise the standard of proof for all the individual tests. Each test is then less likely to produce a false positive and the complete series of analyses will jointly generate a 5 per cent risk.

The usual way to implement the correction is to adjust the critical P value below which we claim statistical significance. This is calculated as:

Critical $P = 0.05/n$

where n is the number of tests to be carried out.

With five tests, we would only declare the result of any individual test to be significant if P was less than $0.05/5 = 0.01$. Under these arrangements, each test will generate only a 1 per cent chance of a false positive and the series of five will entail a 5 per cent risk.

... but it reduces the power of the tests to which it is applied   The Bonferroni correction does a good job of curing the problem it is advertised as fixing – keeping the risk of type I errors down to 5 per cent, but unfortunately it also introduces a new problem. The raised standard of proof required by each individual test increases the chances that a real effect will not be declared significant (more type II errors and therefore reduced power). With the example above, one of the five tests might be for an effect that is genuinely present and it might generate a P value of (say) 0.02. If we had tested for this effect in isolation, we would have used the normal criterion ($P < 0.05$) and we would have obtained a perfectly legitimate significant result. However, once the result is lumped in with four others, it will fail to meet the more demanding Bonferroni corrected target. The greater the number of possibilities

considered, the greater the risk that a real effect will be lost by dilution among a load of irrelevant factors.

 Bonferroni correction – there is no such thing as a free lunch

Keeps the overall risk of any false positives down to 5 per cent by adjusting the level at which P is considered significant.

It also has the unfortunate effect of reducing the power of all tests to which it is applied.

18.3.3 Distinction between primary and secondary (exploratory) analyses

Primary question, primary endpoint and primary analysis   Another way to avoid the hazards of multiple testing is to highlight one particular route through the experimentation and data analysis. Whatever conclusion arises from this route will then be claimed as definitive.

The work may have posed several questions, collected several endpoints and each endpoint may have been subject to more than one statistical analysis. To fully specify a definitive route, we need to specify:

• What is the primary question being asked?

• What will be the primary endpoint that answers that question?

• What will be the primary statistical analysis of that endpoint?

There is then one definitive answer based upon one definitive route and we are guilty of no multiplicity. We can then look at as many additional questions and indulge in as many secondary (or 'exploratory') analyses as we wish. Any conclusions arising from exploratory analyses are subject to all the hazards associated with multiple testing and must be considered highly suspect. Indeed a good way to view such 'conclusions' is that they are not really answers to questions at all, rather they provide guidance as to what might be useful further research. You may see a distinction drawn between 'hypothesis testing' – the role of the primary analysis – and 'hypothesis generation' – the role of secondary analyses.

For example, a primary analysis shows that there is no significant evidence that a medical treatment changes outcomes, but a secondary sub-group analysis suggests that it does produce an effect in younger subjects. In that case, the definitive conclusion would be that the current experiment has not shown an effect. However, the secondary conclusion might provide adequate motivation to repeat the work using only young subjects and for the new experiment, the primary question would become 'does this treatment work in young people?'

To have any legitimacy, the identification of a primary analysis must be finalized before the experimental data have been seen.

🔑 Primary question – primary endpoint – primary analysis

Specify a primary question, primary endpoint and primary analysis of that endpoint. The answer obtained from these can legitimately be claimed as definitive with no contamination by multiplicity.

However, you may also want to take the opportunity to look at several subsidiary questions, which will involve the measurement of additional endpoints. It may then be interesting to carry out all manner of analyses of the various endpoints. Any conclusions thus obtained must be recognized as secondary and tentative. If one of these other conclusions is of particular theoretical or practical importance, it can become the primary question of further research.

The dangers of relying upon the findings of exploratory analyses were nicely summed up by Stephen Senn:

'Enjoy the result you have found by exploratory data analysis, for you will not find it again.'

Fishing trips We could push this idea one stage further and publish indiscriminately (all the data and all the analyses) without any correction for multiple testing, but accept that all conclusions are tentative and should only be used as the basis for hypothesis generation not hypothesis testing.

The collection of masses of data and endless statistical analyses is often referred to derogatorily as a 'fishing trip'. If the authors of this type of work try to pretend that they have produced any reliable conclusions, then they deserve to be pilloried, but so long as they identify their purpose as looking for possible effects that could then be followed up definitively, it is perfectly respectable

18.3.4 Look for patterns of significant results

One thing to check, especially when assessing published data that include multiple testing is whether any apparently significant results form meaningful patterns. Say an author has reported a programme of work that resulted in 30 statistical analyses and has taken no steps to account for multiple testing. We would expect 30 analyses to produce one or two apparently significant results even if there are no real effects present.

If the result is 28 non-significant tests and two 'significant' ones, then it is a nap that these are false positives, meaning absolutely nothing. On the other hand, if there are 25 significant results, it would be churlish to reject all the author's conclusions just because there was multiple testing. It is highly unlikely that such a consistent pattern of significant results would arise by chance and it would have to be accepted that the subject area under investigation must contain real effects. There would still be a danger that an odd false positive might have crept in, and if any particular conclusion was especially critical, it would be useful to check whether it would have survived a Bonferroni correction. If it would not, then it should not be overly relied upon.

⚷ Beware of odd isolated 'significant' results

If multiple tests yield a mass of non-significant results and one or two marginally significant ones, be very suspicious of any claim that the 'significant' ones have any real meaning. If the outcome is a high proportion of significant results, this provides strong evidence, despite the multiple testing.

The other thing to look out for is whether any allegedly significant results make sense in terms of the science underlying the area of investigation. For example, a handful of statistically significant results that form no obvious pattern and which would be difficult to account for on the basis of any known chemical or biological mechanism would not be very convincing, but, if we have a similar number of significant results that all suggest the same sort of effect and if that effect could be readily explained by known mechanisms, these might be taken a lot more seriously.

18.4 The role of scientific journals

If you look through the pirate boxes scattered around this book, you may notice that in a high proportion of cases, the fiddle is worked by seeing the data first and then chopping and changing the analysis until the desired result is obtained. In extreme cases, the process has been memorably referred to as 'the data was tortured until it confessed'.

If those who conduct clinical trials want to be taken remotely seriously by regulatory authorities, they know they will have to record all the main aspects of their proposed trial in advance.

- What question is the trial going to answer?

- What end-point will be used?

- What statistical analysis will be performed?

As a result, most of the pirate boxes have long ceased to be a hazard in clinical trials. Certainly, the real shockers – changing to a one-sided test or selectively reporting the analysis of one sub-group – are dead and buried.

Sadly, academic science and the journals in which it is published fall far short of that standard. How many journals require prior notification of the experiment you are about to perform, analyse and (hopefully) publish? Next time you read an interesting paper, ask yourself a few questions:

- They say the purpose of the experiment was to see if the new process produced harder tablets, but was it really? Maybe they tested six different end-points and only hardness came up as statistically significant.

- It is claimed that 'we planned to test for an increase in fertility and therefore performed a one-sided test'. Did they? Maybe they were looking for a contraceptive effect but found that there were actually more babies and the initial two-sided test produced a P value of 0.07. Was the pirate box at the end of Chapter 10 applied?

- The purpose of the experiment is stated as 'to test whether our new dispensing system increased patient compliance among Bangladeshis aged 27–44 with a severe form of the disease. Really? Could this just possibly be a covert sub-group analysis?

While journals continue to function in their current manner, you may have doubts such as those above, but you will never know. If a minority of journals took the simple precaution of requiring authors to provide prior notification of what they intended to do, the papers they published would be in a different league from the general CV fodder.

18.5 Chapter summary

Unless special precautions are used, multiple testing will increase the risk of generating false positive findings beyond the level of 5 per cent that is normally tolerated.

- Where several treatments are compared against each other, the first step in analysis should be an omnibus test (such as an ANOVA) and, if this proves significant, more detailed analyses can then be undertaken.

- If several endpoints have been determined, a multivariate statistical test should be employed and this can then be followed up by tests concerning the individual endpoints.

- Where an endpoint has been determined on several occasions, a repeated measure ANOVA can be used.

- Data should not be broken down into multiple sub-groups unless either a Bonferroni correction or a distinction between primary and secondary analyses is used to provide additional protection.

The Bonferroni correction raises the standard of proof required for each individual test. This has the effect of maintaining the overall risk of any false positives at 5 per cent, but reduces statistical power.

It is legitimate to declare in advance that the primary purpose of the work is to answer one identified question, and that one specified endpoint and statistical analysis will be used to answer that question. Limitless additional analyses can then be undertaken, so long as any conclusions are recognized as subject to the hazards of multiple testing and cannot be considered definitive.

When authors have used multiple testing, a small number of apparently significant results amid a sea of non-significance should be viewed with suspicion. A high proportion of significant results is, however, more convincing, especially if the significant results form a consistent and logical pattern.

Scientific journals could improve the quality (and possibly the honesty) of data analysis if they insisted on the prior declaration of authors' intentions. Most of the pirate boxes in this book could be abolished overnight.

19
Questionnaires

This chapter will . . .

- Explore the range of data generated by questionnaires

- Give some tips on clear presentation within questionnaires

- Emphasize the need to achieve both an adequate number of completed questionnaires and an adequate rate of completion

- Describe the two stages of analysis – frequency analysis and hypothesis testing

- Describe the difference between planned experimental and epidemiological data

- Describe the problem of confounding in epidemiological data and explain how we reduce the risk of false interpretations

- Emphasize the potential hazard of multiple testing with questionnaire data

Essential Statistics for the Pharmaceutical Sciences   Philip Rowe
© 2007 John Wiley & Sons, Ltd   ISBN 9780 470 03470 5 (HB)   ISBN 9780 470 03468 2 (PB)

19.1 Is there anything special about questionnaires?

Although questionnaires can generally be analysed using techniques that have already been described, they are associated with some distinctive problems and hazards.

19.2 Types of questions

Many text books offer systems for classifying questions. Unfortunately, there seem to be almost as many systems as there are books. I would suggest the following approach, based on the use that will be made of the data.

When we come to analyse the results, we will probably be looking for various possible cause and effect relationships. So let us start by separating those bits of information that are likely to be treated as causes (from here on, I refer to these as 'demographics') from those that are more likely to be seen as effects (referred to as 'outcomes').

19.2.1 Causal factors – 'demographics'

Typically it is things like age, gender, post code, employment, disease status, etc. that are likely to be investigated as possible causal factors influencing outcomes recorded in other questions. It is these that I refer to as 'demographics'.

There is one situation where we would probably avoid the term 'Demographics'. With experimental work such as a clinical trial, the treatment group that a patient belonged to would be the principal causal factor potentially influencing outcomes. However, it would not be customary to consider such data as 'demographics'. Treatment group membership is something to which we allocate subjects, whereas 'demographics' are usually considered to cover pre-existing properties beyond our control.

Collecting respondents' ages   There are not usually too many issues surrounding the gathering of demographic data, but one question that has been put to the author on several occasions is how to collect respondents' ages. The obvious approach is to record the actual numerical ages. However, in further analysis these are often converted into bands (e.g. 16–21, 22–30, 31–45, etc.). There is an argument that, if data are to be analysed in bands, it should be collected in bands. The concern is that, if we collect actual ages and band them later, we could manipulate the choice of bands so as to help obtain a particular result (maybe splitting subjects into above/below 35 failed to produce a significant result, but after trying a few alternatives you discover that splitting into above/below 45 does give statistical significance). This would constitute a form of multiple testing.

However, there is still a strong argument for collecting the actual numerical ages. Once the data are in, you may decide you want to carry out a secondary analysis which requires the ages as a continuous measurement variable. If you only collected ages as bands, you will not have the option.

It is only an opinion, but I would recommend making any decisions about age banding in advance of data collection (to avoid any temptations at a later time), but collect actual ages. That way, secondary analyses requiring numerical ages are still possible. Remember – numerical age data can always be converted to bands, but you cannot reverse the process – actual ages can never be recovered from banded data.

🔑 Recording ages

Suggested approach:

- make decision in advance as to what age bands (if any) will be used;

- collect ages as numerical data.

19.2.2. Outcome data

This can be fairly clearly divided into three types:

- Factual;

- opinion seeking;

- knowledge testing.

Factual questions   Examples include things such as

On how many occasions during the last 7 days did you take pain-killing medicine?

The pain lasted for:

(0–19 min/20 min-1 h/1–3 h/3–6 h/more than 6 h)

Were you able to see a hospital specialist within one calendar month of first seeing your GP? (yes/no)

Opinion seeking questions   These assess more subjective impressions, e.g.

Did you think of the car parking facilities were adequate? (yes/no)

In your opinion the staff were:

(very friendly/friendly/neutral/unfriendly/very unfriendly)

Questionnaires containing opinion-seeking questions are one of the commonest sources of ordinal data. The last example given above would probably be recorded as a score, ranging from (say) 1 (very unfriendly) to 5 (very friendly).

Some investigators like to have an even number of options to avoid a neutral response. If you wanted to force respondents to come off the fence, you could offer the range suggested above, but omitting the option 'neutral'. Then they will have to jump one way or the other – positive or negative.

Knowledge testing questions   Here we are looking to determine how well informed the subject is. We might target either the public (is an educational campaign needed?) or health professionals (in what areas are further training needed?). For example,

What is the normal oral dose of paracetamol for an adult? (10 mg/100 mg/200 mg/1g/5g)

Which one of the following should not be taken with combined oral contraceptives? (paracetamol/rifampicin/vitamin D/lithium/SSRIs)

There may be odd occasions when we only need to find out whether the subject knows a single piece of information and a single question will suffice, but generally we have clusters of such questions to allow a broader test of knowledge.

19.2.3. Closed vs open questions

The form in which questions are posed may be closed or open.

Closed questions   Here the subject is asked to choose from a limited list of possibilities, e.g.

What form of hormone replacement therapy are you presently receiving?

(none/tablets/patches/gel/implant/nasal spray/vaginal ring)'

You will receive a maximum of seven different responses and you know exactly what they will be. Two things need to be ensured:

1. All possibilities are covered.

2. It is clear whether the respondent should select just one option or is free to tick several if appropriate.

Open questions　　These allow free text response, e.g.

　Why did you come to the Accident and Emergency department?'

There is virtually no limit to how many different answers that might elicit!

　Results from closed questions are relatively easy to analyse because the responses are predictable and you can simply count how many choose each option. Analysing responses to open questions is trickier. In the worst case, 100 respondents could produce 100 unique responses. Fortunately things are not generally that bad and certain themes will emerge. You can then count how many raise essentially the same point, without necessarily using identical wording. Such analyses are time-consuming and it is perilously easily to slip into a degree of subjectivity.

　Despite the difficulties, open questions can be valuable:

- They allow respondents to mention aspects that you failed to list in a closed question. You might consider using closed questions as the main data gathering mechanism, but provide an additional, open question such as:

Were there any other reasons why you chose this hospital?

That way, if you forgot to include 'because the next nearest is fifty miles away' in your closed question, the respondent can still raise the issue.

- Open questions can avoid excessive prompting. We might use the following, closed question as a test of knowledge:

The risks of which of the following are reduced by the use of combined oral contraceptives?

(cardiovascular events/ovarian cancer/endometrial cancer/breast cancer/cervical cancer/ pelvic inflammatory disease (PID)/dysmenorrhoea) [You may tick more than one if appropriate.]

This would be a pretty feeble test of knowledge, as all the main issues are listed. If a respondent had completely forgotten that PID was affected, they are going to receive a nice helpful prompt. An open question could ask the respondent to list the appropriate aspects, without providing any prompts.

⚐ Closed and open questions

A mix of closed and open questions will assure access to some data that can be easily and objectively analysed, but also offer the respondent the opportunity to record facts/opinions that you may have accidentally excluded.

19.3 Designing a questionnaire

You do not need to be especially cynical about the human race to know that, if it is possible to misunderstand something, somebody will. Some specific hints to enhance clarity are given below.

19.3.1 Avoid double negatives

The question below is not well worded:

I could not get the tablet container open quickly (yes/no)

The question is phrased in terms of being able to open the container quickly, but a respondent wanting to report that they lacked that ability must select 'yes'. It is all too easy to see the words 'get the container open' and answer 'no' to report your difficulties.
   A better wording would be:

I had difficulty opening the tablet container (yes/no)

The wording is now in terms of 'difficulty' and 'yes' is more obviously the correct way to report problems.

19.3.2 Beware of habituation

It can be a menace when questions include extended blocks that are likely to produce the same answer. After ticking the box for 'yes' for the twelfth question in succession, it is all too easy to switch off all higher intellectual functions and continue repeating the same response, irrespective of the actual questions. Such blocks need to be broken up, to keep the respondent's attention.

19.3.3 Pre-testing

Questionnaires require careful piloting to detect glitches, before we start to use them to generate definitive results. The person who wrote the questions may well think they are unambiguous, but others will still find a way a way to misinterpret them.
   The second great delusion in this area is that you can use a group of your friends to do the piloting. Think about the people who will actually use the questionnaire. Are they as young as your friends? Do they have the same background knowledge? Is their English as good? There is no substitute for doing the job properly and piloting the questionnaire on a sample of individuals from the population you will eventually investigate.

━◯ Careful piloting is vital

You wrote it, so of course you understand it. However, rest assured, somewhere within your masterpiece lurks a question or an instruction that the public will manage to misconstrue. The only way to find it is to try the questionnaire out on a reasonable number of individuals similar to those who will ultimately act as your respondents.

19.4 Sample sizes and return rates

19.4.1. Calculating an appropriate sample size

As with any form of sample-based research, it is important to know in advance how much data (completed questionnaires) will be required. We can calculate a necessary sample size using the approaches described earlier in this book. We just need to identify the primary question, determine what statistical analysis will be used to answer it and then perform a sample size calculation in the normal way.

19.4.2. Beware of self-selected minorities

There is one very large hazard waiting to get you. The danger is that you calculate 100 completed questionnaires are needed, post out 500 and get 110 returned. You have got back more than enough, so what is the problem?

The 110 out of 500 (22 per cent) who did return the questionnaire are a self-selected minority. We already know that they differ in one way – they did return the questionnaire, while the other 78 per cent did not. However, is this decision to complete the form just random or is it linked to other personal characteristics? It would be a brave (foolhardy?) researcher who was prepared to assume that returning or not returning the questionnaire was a purely random choice. The reality is that there are all sorts of ways in which the returners may differ from the non-returners. With a return rate as low as 22 per cent, we could be dealing with a highly unrepresentative minority and any conclusions will be biased towards whatever type of person happens to be most likely to return our questionnaire.

One obvious likelihood is that those with a strong interest in, or opinion concerning, the relevant subject will be more likely to respond. Try asking this in a postal questionnaire:

> Do you believe that corrective laser eye surgery should be provided free by the National Health Service? (yes/no)'

Those who would potentially benefit from free provision could save a huge amount of money, compared with the current situation where most such treatment has to be paid for privately. They will be highly motivated to return the form answering 'yes'. In contrast, anybody who does not need such surgery might gain nothing by its introduction but would also lose very little. To them it would be largely a matter of indifference and they would have little motivation to return the form. The chances are that you will get a low return, almost entirely strongly in favour of the proposal.

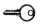 **You need adequate numbers and an adequate return rate**

It is not enough simply to get an adequate *number* of completed questionnaires, it is also vital to obtain a satisfactory return *rate*.

 Show a high level of enthusiasm for your pet topic via a questionnaire with a low return rate

People are unfortunately getting wise to this one, but there is still some mileage left in it.

You want to show that train-spotting is still the UK's number one hobby? Easy. Send out a postal questionnaire that starts with a series of highly technical knowledge-testing questions concerning the wheel configuration of steam engines. Then ask 'how interesting do you find train-spotting?', offering a five-point scale ranging from 'fascinating' to 'utterly boring'. Ninety-five percent of recipients will jib at even attempting to answer the initial questions and bin the whole thing. The handful who survived that obstacle, and therefore have the any real likelihood of returning the questionnaire, will be dedicated train-spotters. Doubtless they will assess their hobby as second to none.

19.4.3. What return rate do we need?

It is impossible to lay down the law about what constitutes an adequate return rate. You would have to consider the potential for bias associated with the particular piece of research. However, once return rates get below about 40 per cent, the onus really is on the researcher to convince his/her readers that the sample is not at risk of bias.

19.4.4. Can we test for a biased return?

Section 19.6.1 will suggest that part of our analysis should routinely be a simple frequency analysis of the demographic data. This may reveal that our sample is biased in terms of gender, age-groups or whatever. However, with very low return rates, it is impossible to be exclude the possibility that our sample may be biased in some way that will not be detected by the demographics we are able to check.

19.5 Analysing the results

Generally the results will be analysed in two stages – frequency analyses and hypothesis testing as described below.

19.5.1 Frequency analyses

This initial stage is a simple reporting of the results for each question in isolation. Some of the questions will produce naturally categorical results and we can simply report the number of respondents who select each possible answer. Gender, occupation, area of residence, etc., fall naturally into this pattern. Other responses such as age, which are essentially continuous variables, may also be broken up into bands as described in Section 19.2.1.

These frequencies serve two possible purposes – they may be of intrinsic interest and they act as checks on your demographics.

Intrinsic interest   Less experienced researchers are surprisingly resistant to the idea that the primary conclusion of a survey can be based upon a simple frequency analysis. Determining the proportion of patients who would prefer to have their drug treatment monitored in a local health centre rather than a hospital or the proportion of people who have various levels of satisfaction with a new service can be perfectly respectable outcomes. The problem is that there are no fancy statistical tests and there can be a sense that something more 'sophisticated' would be of greater merit.

⌐◉ It does not have to be complicated

A simple frequency analysis may be entirely appropriate as the primary outcome of a survey.

Checking demographics   The other key use of frequency analyses is to check that the demographics of a sample are reasonable. If your survey data are supposed to represent all patients being treated at a local health centre, but your frequency analyses reveal that 90 per cent of the responses are from women or there is a similarly disproportionate response from younger people or a particular ethnic group, there are going to be serious questions as to whether your data are credible as a supposedly random sample from the population of service users. If the health centre serves a large new estate full of young families, then you might conclude that a high proportion of younger patients was perfectly reasonable. However, in the absence of such explanations, you may face accusations that you have been selective in questioning certain groups and shunning others.

19.5.2 Hypothesis testing

This is where we start checking whether the answer to one question is linked to the that for another. Examples include:

- Do opinions vary between those who are young/old, male/female, etc.?

- Are knowledge levels greater among those who have received a leaflet than among those who have not?

We will be asking whether any of the outcomes vary according to the demographic or treatment group to which the respondent belongs. Apart from the problem of confounding (see next section), there are no special considerations so far as performing statistical tests is concerned. We just apply the tests outlined in Chapters 6–17. With questionnaires, many outcomes are recorded as simple categorizations – nominal scale data. Consequently questionnaires tend to generate a lot of contingency chi-square tests. Opinions are likely to be recorded on ordinal scales, so questionnaires are an area where non-parametric methods (Chapter 17) are likely to be useful. Interval scale (measured) endpoints are not all that common, and parametric tests (*t*-tests etc.) feature less prominently in questionnaire analysis than in other areas. Scores arising from blocks of knowledge testing questions can be analysed as interval scale data, but they have a nasty habit of forming non-normal distributions, again necessitating a shift to non-parametric alternative tests.

19.6 Confounded epidemiological data

Questionnaires are often used to record epidemiological rather than planned experimental data. To appreciate the difference between these, think about a situation where we want to compare some sort of outcome between smokers and non-smokers.

19.6.1 Planned experimental approach

The planned experimental approach would be to take a group of volunteers, randomly allocate them to smoke or not smoke, leave them to indulge/not indulge for a period of time and then investigate the relevant outcome. From a purely scientific point of view, this approach is impeccable – the inclusion of randomization should ensure that there are no systematic differences between the two groups other than their smoking status and any difference in outcomes can be assumed to be due to smoking.

19.6.2 Epidemiological approach

You might find that your local ethics committee has certain reservations about the above approach, and in practice you would have to make do with an epidemiological study. Here, you simply accept that some folk have already elected to smoke and others not and you look at the relevant outcome in these two pre-existing groups. Your problem now is that people do not just randomly decide whether to smoke. It is very likely that smokers and non-smokers will differ in all sorts of other ways. The smokers may be younger/older, from different social classes, have different patterns of occupation, show a different ethnic mix, etc. So any difference in outcome might be due to smoking, but could also be due to differences in one of these other factors. We say that smoking may be 'confounded' with any of these others factors.

⚷ Confounding

When we create two groups by dividing subjects on the basis of one demographic characteristic, but find the resulting groups also tend to differ in other ways, there is confounding.

19.6.3 An example of confounded factors (age and health)

Assume we investigated attitudes towards a possible change in the supply of emergency (post-coital) contraception. The proposal was that the (then) existing requirement for a prescription should be discontinued, allowing direct supply by a pharmacy. We used a questionnaire to collect a range of demographic data (including age and health status) and also asked simply whether respondents were in favour of, or opposed to, the proposed change.

Our analysis showed that there was an effect of age [see Table 19.1(a)]. Only 26.2 per cent of the older respondents were in favour, vs 74.9 per cent of the youngsters. The results were subjected to a chi-square test and found to be significant. A more conservative view among senior citizens was no great surprise.

What did initially come as a bit of a surprise [Table 19.1(b)] was an additional divide based on health status, with the sick/disabled being less favourable to the proposal than the healthy ($P < 0.001$). However it seemed unlikely that respondents'

Table 19.1 Crude analyses of the influences of age and health status on opinions concerning a liberalized supply of emergency contraception

	Favour	Oppose	Total
(a) Effect of age			
Younger	251 (74.9%)	84 (25.1%)	335 (100%)
Older	123 (26.2%)	346 (73.8%)	469 (100%)
(statistically significant, $P < 0.001$)			
(b) Effect of health status			
Generally healthy	260 (53.8%)	223 (46.2%)	483 (100%)
Chronically sick	114 (35.5%)	207 (64.5%)	321 (100%)
(statistically significant, $P < 0.001$)			

health would be directly linked to views on this issue. What might have happened is that the group with poor health were also generally older than the healthy group, and the more conservative views among the unhealthy respondents was simply a side-effect of that group's generally greater age. If this explanation was correct, it would be a case of confounding between health status and age.

19.6.4 Analysing confounded data

To illustrate how we can tackle this problem, we will continue with the data in Table 19.1.

Refine the data   The secret is to 'refine' the data in order to tease out the individual effects of the two confounded factors. The two parts of table 19.1 are described as 'crude' or 'unrefined' analyses. These terms reflect the fact they potentially confuse the influence of two factors. The intention of Table 19.1(a) is to separate the young from the old, but there is a risk that the young group will also be predominantly healthy while the older group will be relatively sickly. Similarly, the lower table purportedly separates on the basis of health, but may also accidentally produce two groups of unequal age.

   Table 19.1(a) shows 335 younger and 469 older respondents, but each of these contains a mix of healthy and chronically sick individuals. To achieve a refined analysis, we need to further divide each group on health grounds. Table 19.2 shows that the 335 younger individuals can be refined into 260 who are young and healthy and 75 who are young but sickly. The table also reports the numbers favouring/opposing the proposal in each of these more refined groups. The 469 older respondents have been similarly refined.

Analyse the refined data   We can now use the more detailed figures in Table 19.2 to produce refined analyses in which the effects of age and health status are kept distinct from one another. First consider whether age has a truly independent association

Table 19.2   Refining the data

	Favour	Oppose	Total
The 335 younger individuals break down into …			
Younger and generally healthy	197	63	260
Younger and chronically sick	54	21	75
The 469 older respondents break down into …			
Older and generally healthy	63	160	223
Older and chronically sick	60	186	246

with opinion. Table 19.3 shows contingency tables for the possible effect of age, but unlike Table 19.1, we do not leave data for the healthy and sick muddled together – we keep them separate.

We now see the pure effect of age, uncontaminated by variation in health status. Table 19.3(a) still shows a difference in opinion between young and old, and as these are all healthy individuals, the effect can only be due to differences in age. We see the same story in Table 19.3(b) – these are all chronically sick and any difference in opinion can only be attributed to the age difference.

Conclusion: age probably does have a direct effect upon opinion and this is not an artefact of confounding with health status.

We can now try it the other way round – does health status have an independent effect? Table 19.4 investigates the effect of health status after refining for age.

The apparent effect of health status seen in Table 19.1(b) magically evaporates when we refine the data. Within each of these tables, the pattern of opinions for healthy and sickly respondents are virtually identical, so there is no evidence of any independent effect of health status upon opinion.

Conclusion: the apparent effect of health status seen previously was indeed just confounding.

Table 19.3   Refined analyses of the possible effect of age upon opinions on liberalization of supply of emergency contraception

	Favour	Oppose	Total
(a) Generally healthy			
Younger	197 (75.8%)	63 (24.2%)	260 (100%)
Older	63 (28.3%)	160 (71.7%)	223 (100%)
(statistically significant, $P < 0.001$)			
(b) Chronically sick			
Younger	54 (72.0%)	21 (28.0%)	75 (100%)
Older	60 (24.4%)	186 (75.6%)	246 (100%)
(statistically significant, $P < 0.001$)			

Table 19.4 Refined analyses of the possible effect of health status upon opinions on liberalization of supply of emergency contraception

	Favour	Oppose	Total
(a) Younger			
Generally healthy	197 (75.8%)	63 (24.2%)	260 (100%)
Chronically sick	54 (72.0%)	21 (28.0%)	75 (100%)
(statistically non-significant, $P = 0.507$)			
(b) Older			
Generally healthy	63 (28.3%)	160 (71.7%)	223 (100%)
Chronically sick	60 (24.4%)	186 (75.6%)	246 (100%)
(statistically non-significant, $P = 0.342$)			

⚷ **Refine the data**

Where you suspect that an apparent association may be a result of confounding, refine the data to separate the effects of the two factors.

19.6.5 Unrecognized confounding is always a potential problem with epidemiological data

Unfortunately, whenever questionnaires are used to gather epidemiological data (which is much of the time), none of the conclusions ever have the reliability we achieve with planned experiments. In the example we looked at, we had collected data on both of the confounded factors and we could identify and eliminate the problem. However, if we had only gathered data on health status and not recorded respondents' ages, we could well have mistakenly concluded that people's health in some way influenced their opinions.

⚷ **In epidemiological studies, an association is never proof of a cause and effect relationship**

With epidemiological data, always be cautious about ascribing cause and effect relationships. The factor that appears to be having an influence may in fact be confounded with some other unrecognized factor which is the true cause of the particular outcome.

It is wise to look for supporting evidence before interpreting an association as evidence of a cause and effect relationship. In particular, you should be looking for a credible mechanism for any such relationship. Where there is a reasonable biological/chemical/physical explanation for how the alleged causal factor would bring about the effect, you will be on much safer ground.

The classic example is smoking and lung cancer. The initial evidence was necessarily epidemiological and the tobacco barons were long able to muddy the waters with disingenuous arguments that the association might be confounded.

- Maybe there was a gene that tended to make the bearer more likely to choose to smoke and also induced lung cancer.

- People who smoked might also elect to indulge in other activities which were the real cause of the lung cancer.

Now that we can identify the relevant chemicals in cigarette smoke and have elucidated the details of how they damage DNA, the case for a causal relationship is clear to all but a few diehard smokers (there are none so blind as those who do not wish to see).

A commonly used way of side-stepping the issue is to talk in terms of association rather than causality. In the case of the opinions on contraceptive supply, we might have collected data on health status, but not on age. In that case, we would simply be faced with the rather odd fact that those with poorer health generally held more conservative opinions. Recognizing that a cause and effect relationship was unlikely, we could limit ourselves to saying that 'Poor health is associated with a more conservative opinion on changes in the legislation'.

19.6.6 If you're still not convinced, think about this ...

The great example of confounding (OK, it is probably mythical) was the survey that found that people who carried matches were more likely to contract lung cancer – a finding that might be perfectly credible, but needs to be interpreted with caution.

19.7 Multiple testing with questionnaire data

The general problem of multiple testing was covered in the previous chapter. Questionnaires are unfortunately the multiple-tester's happy hunting ground. A questionnaire containing four demographic questions plus three factual, opinion or knowledge testing questions would be a pretty barebones effort (many are far longer). However, with even this minimal example, if we were to take each demographic factor and look to see whether it influenced each of the outcome questions, we would be examining 12 combinations of questions. The chances of obtaining at least one false positive result would exceed 50 per cent. The reality is that most questionnaires present considerably greater temptation than this.

19.7.1 For knowledge testing questions consider basing your primary analysis on an overall knowledge score

One very useful way to reduce multiplicity arises with clusters of knowledge testing questions. If a group of questions all test the same topic, consider combining the results from all the questions to produce an overall score. You can then test whether key demographic factors affect this single result rather than testing each test question separately.

🔑 **Combine a cluster of knowledge testing questions into a single score**

Rather than commit multiple testing by investigating each knowledge testing question separately, carry out a single test on the overall test score.

19.7.2 Identify your primary question in advance

The best defence against multiplicity is to identify, in advance, which potential relationships will be tested for, as primary analyses (as described in the previous chapter). A typical example would be where we have produced a knowledge score and, as a primary analysis, found that two demographic groups scored differently. As a follow-up to this, you might start to ask more detailed questions. For example, did the differences arise because one group was better at answering all the questions or was there just one killer question that one group could answer but the other could not? You could tackle this in a secondary analysis where you would be free to look at individual questions and do as much multiple testing as you wish. The caveat is of course that any conclusions must also be recognized as secondary and not to be relied upon (unless confirmed in subsequent work).

19.8 Chapter summary

The data collected via questionnaires largely fall into two categories – 'demographics' and 'outcomes'. Demographic data describe the basic characteristics of respondents that will commonly be tested for possible causal relationships with the various outcomes.

Although interval scale data (e.g. ages) will probably be reported in bands, there is a good case for collecting it as actual values. Outcome data are commonly classified as 'factual', 'opinion seeking' or 'knowledge testing'.

'Closed' questions have the advantage of bringing only predictable answers that are easily analysed, while 'Open' questions allow respondents to report facts/opinions that might have been excluded by a closed question and they also avoid excessive prompting.

To maximize clarity and minimize errors by respondents:

- avoid double negatives;

- avoid long lists of questions likely to attract the same answer (habituation);

- pre-test the questionnaire on a group of people as similar as possible to the intended target.

An appropriate sample size – number of completed questionnaires – should be calculated (as described in earlier chapters). It is not satisfactory to attempt to compensate for a low return rate by simply increasing the numbers sent out. That tactic risks a biased return.

The first stage in analysing the results is generally a simple frequency analysis – a count of how many respondents produced each possible response, on a question-by-question basis. This information is likely to be of value in its own right and may also alert you to any biases in your sample.

Analysis will then probably progress to hypothesis testing – looking to see whether the answer provided to one question influences the pattern of answers to another question. As so many questionnaire data are nominal scale, contingency chi-tests tend to dominate.

When interpreting your conclusions, it is vital to bear in mind that most questionnaire-based surveys are epidemiological – not planned experiments. Confounding among potential causal factors is rife. The intelligent use of refined analyses will detect some the misleading conclusions that can arise from crude analyses. However, even with this precaution, confounding can still slip through and all epidemiological conclusions need to be treated as provisional.

Endless pairs of questions could be cross-tabulated and questionnaires are a heaven-sent opportunity for multiple testing. Because of this, it is particularly important that the primary analysis is planned in advance. Any amount of secondary analysis can ultimately be performed, so long as it is identified as such.

Part 6
Conclusions

20
Conclusions

Statistics users (and those who teach statistics users) should stop worrying about calculation methods and concentrate on the issues that surround statistical procedures. There is no need for anybody to shy away from statistical testing for fear of hard sums. For simple experimental designs (as advocated later in this chapter), number-crunching is no longer an issue – widely available statistical packages will look after that.

However, statistics users should be attuned to a range of surrounding issues. This book has emphasized five general areas that need attention. Taking these roughly in the order they will be met in the experimental process:

- Be clear about the purpose of the experiment.

- Keep the experimental design simple and therefore clear and powerful.

- Draw up a statistical analysis plan as part of the experimental design.

- Explore the data visually before launching into statistical testing.

- Beware of multiple analyses.

- Interpret both significance and non-significance with care.

20.1 Be clear about the purpose of the experiment

The first step in planning any experimental work should be to clarify exactly what question we are trying to answer.

Essential Statistics for the Pharmaceutical Sciences   Philip Rowe
© 2007 John Wiley & Sons, Ltd   ISBN 9780 470 03470 5 (HB)   ISBN 9780 470 03468 2 (PB)

20.1.1 What sort of question are we posing?

Which of the following questions is your experiment designed to test?

- Do these methods produce different effects?

- Do these methods produce the same effect?

- Does this method produce an effect that at least matches that from another?

As we saw in Chapter 9, each of these questions will lead us into a distinctive statistical approach – difference testing, equivalence testing or non-inferiority testing.

20.1.2 Are we concerned simply with the existence of a difference or is the extent of any difference an issue?

In the case of difference testing, the other question that needs to be settled at a very early stage is whether it would be sufficient simply to know whether a difference exists, or is the size of difference an issue? In some cases the former may be adequate and a simple P value will settle the issue, but where the size of difference is important, the 95 per cent CI for difference must be inspected (see Chapter 9). For equivalence or non-inferiority testing, only the 95 per cent CI is of the slightest use.

20.2 Keep the experimental design simple and therefore clear and powerful

Complex experimental designs looking at the outcomes of several different treatments require analyses of variance (Chapter 13) rather than the simpler t-tests that suffice when just two treatments are considered. A significant outcome from a t-test is open to immediate and unambiguous interpretation, but if any real sense is to be made of a significant ANOVA, it has to be supplemented by some form of follow-up testing. Even after a follow-up test has been applied, the results are still likely to be much less clear-cut than those from a t-test (see for example Figure 13.4). The other big problem with analyses of variance is a loss of power. We saw in Chapter 13 that the difference between two treatments may emerge as statistically significant so long as we restrict ourselves to comparing just those two, but if we throw in additional treatments they may dilute the contrast with a loss of statistical significance.

A similar pattern emerged with contingency chi-square tests (Chapter 16). The simplest 2×2 tables led to clear unambiguous conclusions while results from larger tables were much less easily interpreted.

20.3 Draw up a statistical analysis plan as part of the experimental design – it is not a last minute add-on

Even the least pernickety experimenter recognizes that all the basic details of laboratory procedures have to be planned well before putting hand to test-tube and yet it seems normal practice (especially among academics) that statistical analysis is the merest after-thought. The author recently reviewed a protocol for a postgraduate project that blithely asserted 'when all the data have been collected, a statistician will be consulted to show the results are significant'.

In this book there are references to a whole range of reasons to avoid late arrival at the statisticians' ball. The author has personal experience of some colleague or other falling foul of all the following pitfalls.

20.3.1 Inadequate power

The experiment is done, the analysis is non-significant and it now emerges that the experiment was so underpowered that it was a waste of time doing it. How many times have we been there? If statistical issues had been considered from the start, there would (hopefully) have been a timely consideration of this aspect

20.3.2 Poor experimental design

The efficiency of an experiment can depend crucially on the details of its design. A classic example is whether to design a paired or unpaired study. We saw in Chapter 12 that a paired experiment followed by a paired t-test may be much more powerful than the unpaired equivalent. In some circumstances, the difference is so great that an unpaired design could be predicted to have inadequate power, leading to inevitable failure. In other cases, the difference in power may less dramatic and you could waste your time struggling with the extra practical complexities of a paired design.

20.3.3 Unanalysable results

I remember a colleague approaching me with the finished results of a large experiment, with an unusually complex design that was supposed to focus on one experimental factor but also dragged in a range of secondary matters. Needless to say, I had not been asked to play any role in planning the work, but being soft, I agreed to try to analyse the results. It was a real struggle and in particular I could not figure out a satisfactory test for the effect of the main experimental factor. It eventually emerged that hidden within this monster there was no satisfactory control data for the main factor.

Strictly speaking, this error should have been identifiable even without prior planning of the statistical analysis. However, if the stats had been planned in advance, it would have provided a reliable last line of defence against such disasters.

20.3.4　Optimal analysis no longer acceptable

We have already seen that some statistical approaches are perfectly acceptable so long as full details are declared in advance. For example:

- setting the limits of equivalence (Chapter 9);

- one-tailed testing (Chapter 10);

- follow-up tests for ANOVAs (Chapter 13);

- division of the outcomes of multiple analyses into primary and secondary conclusions (Chapter 18).

All of these techniques enhance analysis in one way or another, but none of them can legitimately be employed if they were not planned in advance of seeing the data.

🔑 The 90 per cent: 10 per cent rule

For most experiments, 90 per cent of the statistical work should be done before data collection and 10 per cent afterwards.

- Before – identify the primary question, primary end-point and primary statistical analysis; establish equivalence limits where necessary; perform power and sample size calculations.

- After – carry out the planned analysis.

20.4　Explore your data visually before launching into statistical testing

One of the draw-backs of modern statistical packages is that analyses are almost too easy to execute. It is tempting to go straight from data acquisition to t-test with no further thought. However, many an embarrassment can be avoided by spending a few minutes exploring your data visually before plunging into formal tests.

20.4.1 Is your data normally distributed?

Figures 17.1 and 17.2(a) used either a scatter diagram or histogram to expose the non-normal distribution of toxic metabolite production and warned us that the direct application of a *t*-test was hazardous, whereas Figure 17.2(b) provided reassurance that log transformation had pretty much fixed the problem. Just by looking at Figure 17.4, we knew immediately that there was little point even trying to transform the analgesic effectiveness scores to normality; we were better off just going straight to a non-parametric test.

20.4.2 Inspect the variability in the data

From Figure 12.1 it was clear that variability among subjects' weights was much greater than that among the changes in their weights. Consequently, a paired *t*-test was always going to be much more powerful than the two-sample version.

20.4.3 How are we going to proceed if there is significant evidence of interaction in a two-way analysis of variance?

If you just dive into a two-way analysis of variance and obtain significant evidence of interaction, how are you going to interpret it? If you had already plotted a graph such as Figure 13.6, you would know that what we are seeing is reasonably benign quantitative interaction. That would re-assure us that it is OK to make blanket statements such as 'increased compression force will produce higher strength tablets'. However, if your graphical exploration of the data produced something like Figure 13.8, you would be forewarned to avoid such generalizations.

20.4.4 Is there clear evidence of nonlinear relationships?

Before attempting correlation analysis or the production of a regression equation, use a simple graph to check that you are not dealing with an obviously nonlinear relationship. If you obtain a graph such as Figure 14.7, you can proceed to such techniques with confidence, but Figure 14.6 (c, d or e) would warn you not to be so silly.

20.5 Beware of multiple analyses

As we saw in the last chapter, multiple testing can incur far more than the standard 5 per cent risk of making a false positive claim.

Do not do it yourself. People thrash around analysing and re-analysing the data – swapping from parametric to non-parametric, making a last minute switch to a one-sided test, fishing out a sub-set that suits their purposes. You may manage to squeeze out a barely significant *P* value, but if the finding is anything other than trivial, it will probably end up being exposed as a false finding and you will just look silly.

Do not let other people get away with it. Ask awkward questions. Was that really the question they set out to answer? How many other end-points did they measure? Does it really seem credible that they would have committed to a one-sided test before seeing the data?

20.6 Interpret both significance and non-significance with care

Throughout the book (and especially in Chapter 11) it has been emphasized that the achievement of statistical significance does not provide indisputable evidence of an experimental effect. What it does show is that we should give greater credence to claims of an experimental effect. In cases where prior evidence or general scientific principles already suggest an effect to be likely, the new evidence will leave us pretty convinced of its presence. Where an effect would be contrary to all science and logic, a significant result would dilute our scepticism, but not overthrow it in a single step.

Of course, having read Chapter 9, you will not fall into the trap of confusing statistical significance with practical significance.

In the case of non-significance, the interpretation depends upon background events. If we went into the experiment simply looking for a difference and have not given the matter further thought, then we are at a dead-end. No effect has been shown, but sadly neither can we can claim to have shown the absence of an effect. If we had had the foresight to establish equivalence limits before performing the experiment, a demonstration that there is no effect of practical consequence may be possible.

Index

95% confidence interval, *see* confidence
    interval
Ages, 258–9
Alpha, 76
Alternative hypothesis, 70–1
Analyses, 252–72
    exploratory, 252–3
    optimal, 280
    primary, 252–3, 272
    secondary, 252–3, 272
    of variance, 145–68
Analysis of variance, one-way, *see* One-way
    analysis of variance
Analysis of variance, two-way, *see* Two-way
    analysis of variance
ANOVA, *see* Analyses, of variance
Arithmetic mean, 64

Balanced samples, 107, 155, 160–1
Beta, 90–1
Bias, 37–8
Bimodal data, 16
Bonferroni correction, 251–2

Calibration, 183–5
Centiles, 23
Central tendency, 10–16
Chi-square, 202–19
    test, contingency, *see* Contingency
        chi-square test
    test, goodness-of-fit, *see* Goodness-of-fit
        chi-square test
    critical values for, 205

Coefficient of variation, 19–20
Confidence interval, 50
    for difference between means, 60–1, 72–3
        calculation of, 61
        variation in sample size, 61
        variation in standard deviation, 61
    for difference between proportions,
        213–14
    for mean, 49–60, 137
        calculation of, 52–53
        Excel, 53
        meaning of, 51
        one-sided, 57–60
            calculation of, 58–9
            Excel, 58
            presenting visually, 59
        presenting visually, 53
        reliability of, 53–4
        requirement for normal distribution,
            61–5
        variation in level of confidence, 51–2,
            55–6
        variation in sample size, 52, 55
        variation in standard deviation, 52, 54–5
    for proportion, 199–200
        calculation of, 199–200
Confounding, 266–71
Contingency chi-square test, 211–19
    factors affecting, 211–12
    null hypothesis for, 211
    performing, 212–13
    sample size for, 217–19
    Yates correction, 212–13

Essential Statistics for the Pharmaceutical Sciences Philip Rowe
© 2007 John Wiley & Sons, Ltd

Contingency table, 210
  2×2, 214
  larger, 214–17
  sub-division of, 216
Continuity, 205, 212
Continuous measurement data, *see* Interval
    data
Correlation, 170–78
  cause and effect relationships, 177–8
  coefficient, 170–1
  negative, 170
  Pearson, 171
  positive, 170
  Spearman, *see* Spearman correlation
  test, 172–7
    factors affecting, 173–4
    non-linearity, 175–6
    null hypothesis for, 172
    performing, 176–7

Data, 3–6
  balanced, 155
  bimodal, 16
  continuous, 4
  discontinuous, 4–6
  epidemiological, 266–7, 270–1
  interval, 4
  nominal, 4, 197–208, 210–19
  ordinal, 4, 233–5, 237–41
  paired, 133
  polymodal, 14, 29
  refinement of, 268–70
  skewed, 224–6
  trimodal, 16
  types, 3–6
  unimodal, 14
Deciles, 23
Demographics, 258–9, 265
Descriptive statistics, 9–26
  calculation, 23–5
    with Excel, 23–4
    with Minitab, 24
    with SPSS, 24
Design of experiments, 140–1, 156, 164–5
  full factorial, 156
  multi-factorial, 164–5
  paired, 140

  advantages of, 140
  disadvantages of, 140–41
Deviation, standard, *see* Standard deviation
Difference testing, 107, 110
Dispersion, 16–20, 22
Distribution, 27–34
  free tests, 232–3
  non-normal, 28–31
  normal, *see* Normal distribution
  polymodal, 29
  skewed, *see* Skewness
  truncated, 30–1
Dunnett's test, 152, 250
  level of confidence, 154
  performing, 154–5

Epidemiology, 266–7, 270–1
Equivalence, 105–12
  limits, 105–15
  testing, 107–11
    incorrect, 110–11
  zone, 105–15
    equivalence testing, 108–9
    non-inferiority testing, 112
    practical significance, 106–7
Error, 76, 90–1, 154
  rate, test wide, *see* test wide error rate
  sampling, *see* sampling error
  type I, 76
  type II, 90–1
Expected frequencies, 203–4, 206–7
Exploratory analyses, 252–3
Extrapolation, 182–3

Factors, 146, 156
Failure zone, 112–3
False negative, 90–1
False positive, 75–6
Fishing trips, 253
Follow up tests, 151–5
Frequency analyses, 265–6
Full factorial design, 156

General linear model, 161
Geometric mean, 64
Goodness-of-fit chi-square test, 202–7
  calculation of, 203–7

expected frequencies, 203–4, 206–7
  null hypothesis for, 203
  performing, 203–7
  Yates correction, 205–6

Habituation, 262
Hypothesis, 70–1
  alternative, 70–71
  generation, 252
  null, 70
  test, 68, 252, 266–72

Independent samples t-test, *see* two-sample
    t-test
Indicators, 10–22
  of central tendency, 10–16
  of dispersion, 16–20, 22
Interaction, 157–9, 160, 161–4
  qualitative, 161–4
  quantitative, 163–4
Interpolation, 183
Inter-quartile range, 22
Interval data, 4

Journals, 126, 254

Kruskal-Wallis test, 237–9
  follow up tests for, 239
  performing, 238–9

Least squares fit, 179–80
Levels, 146, 156
Limits of equivalence, 105
Log transform, *see* Transform, log

Mann-Whitney test, 228–31
  interpretation of significance, 230–1, 243
  null hypothesis for, 231
  performing, 230
  ties, 229, 230
Mean, 10–11
  arithmetic, 64
  calculation of, 11
  geometric, 64
Median, 11–14
  calculation of, 12, 13
Mode, 14–16

Multi-factorial design, 164–5
Multiple regression, *see* regression, multiple
Multiple testing, 147, 191, 247–55, 271–2,
    281–2
  end points, 249–50
  subsets, 249–50
  time points, 249
  treatments, 248, 250
Multivariate statistics, 250

Negative, false, 90–91
Ninety-five per cent confidence interval, *see*
    confidence interval
Nominal data, 4, 197–208, 210–19
  inefficiency of, 200–1, 207
Non-inferiority testing, 111–13
Non-parametric methods, 228–42
Non-significance, 75, 282
Normal distribution, 27–34, 61–3, 224–6
  proportions within limits, 31–4
Normal range, 33
Null hypothesis, 70

Omnibus tests, 250
One-sided interval, 57–60
One-sided testing, 117–26, 143
One-tailed testing, *see* one-sided testing
One-way analysis of variance, 146–56
  balanced data, 155
  factors affecting, 149–50
  multiplicity of t-tests, 147
  null hypothesis for, 148–9
  performing, 150–1
  practical significance, 153
  requirements for, 155–6
Ordinal data, 4, 233–5, 237–41

P values, 83–8, 113–15
  extreme, 86
  reporting, 86
Paired data, 133
Paired design, *see* design, paired
Paired t-test, 133–44
  applicability, 139–40
  equivalence testing, 142–3
  factors affecting, 138–9
  non-inferiority testing, 142–3

Paired t-test (*continued*)
  null hypothesis for, 136
  one-sided, 143
  performing, 136–8
  power, 139–40
  practical significance, 142–3
  requirements for, 141
  sample size calculation, 142
Parametric methods, 224
Pearson correlation, 171
Piloting, 262–3
Plan for statistical analysis, 279–80
Point estimate, 50
Polymodality, 14, 29
Population, 35–6
Positive, false, 75–6
Power, 91–4, 97
  curve, 91–3
Practical significance, *see* significance,
  practical
Prediction by regression, 182
  reverse, 183–5
Pre-testing of questionnaires, 262–3
Primary analyses, 252–3, 272
Proportions, 198–208, 210–19
  confidence interval for, 199–202
  factors affecting precision, 198–9,
    201–2

Quantiles, 22–3
Quartiles, 20–2
  calculation of, 20
Questionnaires, 257–73
  design of, 262
  frequency analyses, 265–6
  hypothesis testing, 266–72
  multiple testing, 271–2
  pre-testing, 262–3
  refinement of data, 268–70
  return rates, 263–4
  sample sizes, 263–4
Questions, 259–60
  closed, 260–1
  factual, 259
  knowledge testing, 259–60
  open, 260–1
  opinion seeking, 259–60
Quintiles, 23

R-square, 181, 190–1
Random sampling error, *see* Sampling error,
  random
Range, normal, 33
Ranking, 12, 228–30, 240–1
Rates of return, 263–4
Refinement of data, 268–70
Regression, 178–92
  equation, 180, 185, 186
  least squares fit, 179–80
  line of best fit, 179
  multiple, 185–91
    equation, 186, 189–90
    forward selection of predictors, 189
    performing, 187–9
    prediction of dependent variable, 190
    removal of predictors, 188–9
    R-square, 190–1
  null hypothesis for, 182
  performing, 181–2
  prediction, 182–5
    extrapolation, 182–3
    interpolation, 183
    reverse, 183–5
  reverse prediction, 183–5
  R-square, 181, 190–1
Repeated measures ANOVA, 251
Return rates, 263–4
Reverse prediction, 183–5
Robustness, 13, 22, 61–2, 79, 224

Sample, 35–46
  size calculation, 94–101
Sampling error, 37–42, 198–201
  interval data, 37–42
  nominal data, 198–201
  random, 38–9
    factors governing, 39–42
    sample size, 40–1
    variability of data, 41–2
Secondary analyses, 252–3, 272
SEM, 42–6
  calculation of, 44–6
    Excel, 46
    Minitab, 46
    SPSS, 46
  definition of, 43–4
  variation in sample size, 44–5

variation in SD, 44–5
Significance, 74–5, 85, 282
  meaning of, 127–32
  practical, 104–7, 142–3, 153
  statistical, 104, 106, 127–32
Simplicity of design, 278
Skewness, 29–30
  negative, 29–30
  positive, 29–30
Spearman correlation, 171, 239–42
  coefficient, 241
  performing, 240–1
Standard deviation, 16–20
  calculation of, 18
  units of, 19
Standard Error of Mean, *see* SEM
Statistical analysis plan, 279–80
Statistical significance, *see* significance,
    statistical
Statistics descriptive, *see* Descriptive
    statistics
Student's t-test, *see* two-sample t-test
Sub-group analyses, 248–50

Tables, contingency, *see* contingency tables
Test wide error rate, 154
Testing, 72–3
  difference, 107
  equivalence, 110–11
  multiple, *see* multiple testing
  non-inferiority, 111–13
  one-sided, 117–26
Ties, 229, 239
Transform, 63–5, 224–8
  log, 63–5, 224–8
  square, 65
  square-root, 65
Trimodality, 16
t-tests, 67–144
  paired, *see* paired t-test
  two sample, *see* two-sample t-test
Tukey's test, 152–4, 250
  level of confidence, 154
  performing, 152–3
Two-sample t-test, 67–126
  balanced, 107
  factors affecting, 76–9
  log transform, 224–8

null hypothesis, 70
one sided, 117–26
  abuse of, 121–4
  null hypothesis for, 118–19
  performing, 119–120, 125
  protocol, 124–5
  risk of false positive, 120–1
performing, 72–3
power, 93–4
practical significance, 104–7
requirements for, 79–80
risk of false positive, 75–6
sample size calculation, 95–101
  factors affecting, 95–101
  Minitab, 98
  performing, 98
  SPSS, 98
significance, 73–5
Two-way analysis of variance, 156–64
  balanced data, 160–1
  factors, 156
  interaction, 157–9, 160, 161–4
    graphical check for, 158–9
  interpretation, 160
  levels, 156
  null hypotheses for, 159
  performing, 159–60
Type I error, 76
Type II error, 90–1

Unimodality, 14

Variables, 178
  dependent, 178, 181, 183–5
  independent, 178, 181, 183–5
Variation, 16–20
  coefficient of, 19–20
  inter-group, 149
  intra-group, 149
Visual analogue scale, 30
Visualisation of data, 280–1

Web site, xv, xviii
Welch's approximate t, 80
Wilcoxon paired samples test, 236–7

Yates correction, 205–6, 212–13

Zone of equivalence, *see* Equivalence zone